Clinical Social Work with Latinos in New York-USA

Author:

César M. Garcés Carranza, PhD.

Ordering Information:

For orders and inquiries, please contact:
1-888-404-1388
www.goldtouchpress.com
book.orders@goldtouchpress.com

Printed in the United States of America

Dedication

To

My family

ACKNOWLEDGEMENT

I wish to express my gratitude and deepest thanks to my wife Ellen and our daughter Rachel who made a unique contribution to this endeavor.

"A people without the knowledge of their past history, origin and culture is like a tree without root"-

Marcus Garvey

TABLE OF CONTENTS

Clinical Social Work Interventions with Latinos in New York , USA

Introduction:

To talk about mental health in the Latino community in New York is considered a taboo. This implies that parents, children, and schoolteachers do not talk enough about this issue. Some people consider it inappropriate to talk about mental health problems outside of the household.

The author's experiences practicing clinical social work with Latinos and people from other minority groups in New York is extensive. He tries to describe the actual context of clinical social work with Latinos in New York, describing the principal areas of the professional practice and the needed education to practice this specialty. The main points of this personal exploration rests in a reflection that tries to explain the advantages of being a bilingual, bicultural clinical social worker. Finally, will make recommendations and suggestions for the Latin American social work movement that has been growing up for the last few years.

As a way of invitation, clinical social workers should contribute to initiatives of research, not only to prove their effectiveness in their therapeutic interventions, but also to promote the recognition and acceptance of other social work colleagues in the field of health and mental health. Clinical social workers should understand that they play a key role finding and treating a series of mental health problems, which encompasses from the post-traumatic stress to the emotional reactions that people suffer when they face problems related to mental health. As a profession that is based on human rights, the specialty of clinical social work has an essential function in all societies, easing the communities to raise their voice and defend their rights along with others. The power of clinical social work rest in its own professional foundation, which implies its capacity to create a participatory democracy, to link communities in sustainable futures and protecting human rights.

Key words:

Social work, clinical social work, psychiatric social work, Latino, mental health, community mental health clinics, hospital, stigma., culture.

For the past 36 years Dr. Garcés has been practicing as a clinical social worker in the hospital setting (emergency room, intensive care units, medical surgical units, discharge planning), and in community outpatient psychiatric clinics in the in the State of New York, with people from different social, ethnic, and multicultural backgrounds, especially with the Latin American communities. As a clinical social worker, he can find the major psychosocial and emotional problems, including crisis interventions, providing counseling, and exploring alternatives to find and apply alternatives to face emotional problems such as depression and anxiety. Restoring the functioning throughout implementation of a plan of action and providing adequate interventions to people with mental health problems is part of his daily practice in community mental health clinics. The focus of his interventions is the basis of his concentration of what happens in *"the here and now"* and not in the past.

Mental health as part of the overall health of people, is a part of human growth and therefore of the development of nations. Mental health is not only based on subjective conditions; it is also based on objective conditions. A comprehensive look at this statement assumes an understanding of mental health as an element that is inserted in the society. Mental health is related to the deployment of different human abilities in different moments of life, the things that we do, be them small or big. It involves building and developing active links that are reality transformers, which allows us to take care of our personal needs and psychic well-being as well as that of others.

Social work is a profession and academic discipline that is committed to improve the social and emotional well-being of people, changes, and social justice. This profession works towards research and practice to improve the quality of life of people, groups, and the community where they live. Social work develops interventions through research, administration, local community organizations, direct practice, prevention, and education. Often, research is focused in areas such as human development, mental health, public administration, evaluation of programs and community development. Social workers are organized in local professional, national, and international groups. Social work is an interdisciplinary field that includes theories of economics, education, sociology, medicine, philosophy, and anthropology (NASW, 2012).

To talk about mental health among Latinos in New York, is also to talk about poverty, stigma, and inequality. The present situation of mental health is an important indicator of the actual conditions of most of the Latino population. This offers a distinctive look at living in poverty, exclusion, and inequality that our society goes and should be taken care as a part of a comprehensive strategy against poverty.

What is Culture?

The term was first used by the Pioneer English Antropologist Edward B. Tylor in his book, Primiutive Culture, published in 1871. Tylor said that culture is "that complex whole which includes knowledge, beleif, art, law, morals, custom, and any other capabilities and habits acquired by man as a member of society." It is not limited to men. Women possess and créate it as well.

Culture is a powerful human tool for survival, but it is a fragile phenomenon. It is constantly changing and easily lost because it exists only in our minds. Our written languages, governmentrs, buildings, and other man-made things are merely the producto of culture (Tyler, 1871; Melvine. L. M., 2012).

Subculture:

Subculture is often defined as the beliefs and attitudes that separate groups within the same broad culture. As a layer of subculture, is often made up of differences in religioin, socioeconomic status, and even race. Americans are very familiar with subcultures. One needs only to spend a day in New York City to experience the subcultures of places like Little Italy, El Barrio, China Town. Many of thespeople in these neighborhoods share the national culture of being Americans, but they may differ in how they dress, what they eat, and how they worship (Dresser, W.,2017).

Layers of Culture:

There are three layers of culture that are part of a learned behavior patterns and perceptions. Most obviously is the body of cultural traditions that distinguish a specific societrty. When people speak of Italian, Spanish, Italian, or Japanese culture, they are referring to the shared language, traditions, and beleifs that set each of these peoples apart fro others. In miost cases, those who share a culture do so because they adquired it as they were raised by parents and other family members who have it.

The second layer of culture that may be parto f our identity is subculture. In complex, diverse societies in which people have come from different parts of the world, they often retain mucho f their original cultural traditions. As a result, they are likely to be parto f an identifiable subculture in their new society. The shared cultural traits of subcultures set them apart from the resto f their society.Examples of identifiable subcultures in the United States include ethnic groups such as African Americans, Mexican Americans, and Latin Americans. Me=,bers of each of each of these subcultures share a common identity, food tradition, dialect language, and other cultural traits that come from their common ancestral background and experience. As the cultural differences between members of a suubculture and the dominant national culture blur and eventually disapear, the subculture ceases to exist except as a group of people who claim a common ancestry.

The third layer of culture consist of cultural universals. These are learned behavior patterns that are shared by al lof humanity collectivelly. No matter where people live in the world, they share these universals traits (Dresser, W., 2017).

Examples of human cultural traits:

1. Communicating with verbal language consisting of limited set of sounds and gramatical rules for constructing sentences.
2. Using age and gender to classify people (e.g., teenager, senior citizen, woman, man).
3. Classifying people base don marriage and descent relationships and having kinship terms to refer to them (e.g., wife, mother, uncle, cousin).
4. Raising children in some sort of family setting.
5. Having sexual división of labor (e.g., men's work vs. Women's work).
6. 6. Having concept of privacy.
7. 7. Having rules to regulate sexual behavior.
8. 8. Distinguishing between Good and bad behavior.
9. 9. Having some sort of body ornamentation.
10. Making jokes and playing games.
11. Having art.
12. Having some sort of roles for the implementation of community decisions.

Culture and Society:

Culture and society are not the same thing. While cultures are complexes of learned behavior patterns and preceonceptions, societies are groups of interacting organisms. Societies are groups of people who directly or inderictly interact with each other (Tyler, E. B., 1871).

Cultural concepts:

The author's daily activities with clients/patients and families who only speak Spanish in a State where the dominant language is English, shows an understanding about the complexity of the emergency room which is the entrance to the hospital system. These experiences can also be extended to patients and families of countries of different languages. Those social workers who do not have knowledge of the Spanish language, often have difficulty in communicating with clients/patients and their families. The author's experience in the hospital setting is extensive. He has worked at the Bronx Lebanon Hospital Center, Bronx, New York for over two decades (1989-2013), and by being admitted to a hospital when he first arrived at the United States and did not speak English. He was interviewed by doctors and nurses who did not speak Spanish, and with the help from a translator who also did not speak his language. As a result of this, the translator did not understand what he said and gave incorrect information to the doctor who was examining him. Therefore, it is very well understood the problems that clients/patients face when they are interviewed by people who do not speak their language. According to Campinha-Bacote (1998), cultural competence is about cultural knowledge, attitudes, behavior and including politics that train professionals to be able to function in different intercultural contexts.

As the United States changes into a diverse racial, multicultural, and ethnical country, social workers need to understand the different ethnical perspectives, cultural and values of people to whom they provide their professional services. Lack of knowledge and the understanding of social and cultural differences could end up in negative consequences for people from diverse cultural and ethnic groups. An adequate intervention is needed for social workers to respect and to not judge people who need their professional intervention.

This implies respect for the belief about health and mental health problems, as well as the solution of a problem that is presented by the client/patient. Cultural competence in this area of intervention requires general knowledge of aid, actions that are common in society, the institutions involved, they are culturally separated, which could be difficult for an adequate intervention, or could be that the services being offered are culturally inadequate or they are not available. The administrators of hospitals and community mental health centers should develop strategies to hire, keep, and promote within these institutions, teams of diverse multicultural professionals who are competent in the areas where they provide professional services. By doing so, clients/patients could efficiently communicate in their language. Social workers work with people who do not have power or influence. For this reason, it is important to examine issues of oppression, and social workers need to be culturally competent.

Without cultural awareness, clinical social workers contribute to the oppression when working with client/families from other cultures or ethnic backgrounds. This is unethical practice and can cause client/patients great harm (Sue,D., Arredondo, P., Mc Davis, R., 1992). Clinical social workers need skills to assess clients' entire system. If ignored, social workers may echo society's oppression by assuming that client's/patients need to change, rather than working for societal change (Pinderrhughes, E. 1989).

To build competent community mental health centers, means changing beliefs about other cultures or ethnic groups, and how they communicate and work. This means that the structure, leadership, and activities of an organization should reflect the values, perspectives, lifestyle, and people's priorities. Because social changes are happening fast, organizations are beginning to understand the need to hire professionals who are cultural and ethnically competent. Social workers must be aware that, if they do not improve their skills , the profession will be paralyzed as a professional organization.

The present hostile political climate of the United States may cause fear, anxiety, depression, and toxic stress among the Latino population and other minority groups. Intimidation, bullying and hostility in the schools, may also cause stress among Latino and other minority students. The salary discrepancy along with the use of social networks and their complexity of how they affect the mental health is also a crucial factor. According to experts of mental health, stress is not the only principal cause of emotional problems, but it can contribute to worsen the need for people with these conditions to control their mental health. Even though clinical social workers treat these types of emotional problems, Latinos, as a group have less probability of access to mental health services, especially children and young adults.

The modern clinical social worker must adapt to the world globalization where institutions are having an impact on the rules and unilateral practices. The progressive increase of social culturally different consumers, especially in hospitals and community mental health centers, constitute a challenge for clinical social workers. The National Association of Social Workers (NASW, 2001), defines social work as "a profession that promotes social changes, solutions to human relationships and empowers people to improve their social wellbeing." By using theories of human behavior and social systems, social workers intervene in places where people relate to their social environment. The principles and human rights are fundamentals for clinical/psychiatric social work.

The assertion of a group of social work representatives around the world clearly asserted that the element that encompasses the modern practice of this profession are interrelated within the outside world and the internal psychological experiences of the individual. To better understand how to be able to help under these circumstances, social workers must develop the ability to assess and to intervene in various places with individuals, families, and with groups of people from different ethnic and cultural groups. Such interventions must be understood within the legal functional context, needs of services for the consumers, and with the firm foundation against racism and discrimination. The borders between countries are diminishing because of economic pressures, geopolitics, regions, wars, internal and ethnic conflicts that provoke, among other things, migrations. That is why cultural competency in clinical social work is a need and expectation of all public services that reflects the multicultural increase in a diverse society, country, or region where we live (Walker, S., & Beckett, C., 2005).

Certain types of connotative languages could be ambivalent, causing misunderstandings that could scare the client/patient, as well as the family. Because of this, the clinical social worker, the client/patient, and family members could end up in conflictive situations. There is a need for the communication to be clear and adequate between the clinical social worker and the client/family. Language obstacles could be overcome when the social worker speaks the same language of the client/patient and family members. Communication is not easy, even when people have the same history of experiences and shared values or speak the same language. There are situations when couples have been living for over thirty years and still have misunderstandings. It is no surprise, therefore, to find lack of communication among people who do not know each other. Whatever is said could be heard in a unique way by the other person or it also could be misunderstood.

Lumb, D. (1999), defines cultural competence as "the group of knowledge and skills that the social worker and other health care professionals have to be able to be competent multicultural with clients." Clinical social work deals with different components of culture, which include gender, race, sexual orientation, religion, etc. Green, J. (1999), author of *"Cultural Awareness in the Human*

Services," was certain when he said that the practice of cultural competence must have knowledge base, professional training, and proper interventions to be able to understand people of diverse cultures and ethnic groups. Betancourt, J. R (2001), also mentioned that culture is a group of learned beliefs, shared values, styles of living and communication, practice, costumes, and points of view on what has to do with functions and social relationships.

Not everybody who speaks Spanish are the same. On the contrary, these people have different social histories, values, cultural and religious costumes. The countries of Spanish speaking population are geographically different. They have specific costumes as well as ethnic and cultural blends. The people from Latin America are associated with nineteen countries of Spanish speaking language, in the Caribbean, Central and South America. The following countries are: Cuba, Dominican Republic, Puerto Rico, Costa Rica, El Salvador, Nicaragua, Panamá, Guatemala, Honduras, México, Bolivia, Paraguay, Uruguay, Ecuador, Venezuela, Colombia, Chile, Perú, and Argentina. The exception is Brazil where the official language is Portuguese.

When the clinical social worker is from a country different than the ethnic group of the client/patient, misunderstandings are common. The clinical social worker who lacks knowledge of the language of the client/patient must be careful and avoid making false assumptions about the expectations of the treatment that will be offered. The clinician and the client/patient bring their own social and cultural patterns to the experience of the interview, which must be at once solved, to be able to get equal access and quality of treatment services.

During an interview, a client/patient with a clinical social worker of different ethnicity may assume that the clinician will not understand his/her problem. These could decrease the likelihood that the client/patient will continue services. The opposite is also true. Some clinical social workers have a poorer opinion of those clients/patients whom they see as having significantly different views from themselves (Davis, L., Proctor, E., 1989).

Latin American ethnicity:

"Latino" defines a cultural or ethnic group, not a racial category. It is the population's diversity. Despite many differences, Latinos share cultural characteristics, such as importance of family, strong feelings of support to one's family, obedience. Family also includes nuclear family, extended family, friends who have strong bonds to the family.

Machismo is a term used to describe the belief that men are to be providers and it is their duty to keep families safe (Comas-Diaz, L., 1995). According to Anderson. S., Sabatelly, R. (1999). Marianismo is an aspect of the female gender role in Hispanic American folk cultures, strictly intertwined with machismo and Roman Catholicism (Stevens, E. P., 1973). It revolves around the veneration for feminine virtues like interpersonal harmony, inner strength, self-sacrifice, family, chastity, and morality among Latino women. According to Anderson, S., Sabatelli, R. (1999), The degree of machismo and marianismo present within families varies. These roles influence family dynamics and need to be considered during social work interventions. Comas-Diaz, L. (1995), argues that Puerto Rican women may display marianismo at home and hembrismo at work. This awareness can help clinical social workers understand contradictory behavior (Comas-Diaz, L. 1995).

Cultural competence:

There is a need for an open communication with client/patients to avoid misunderstandings. language obstacles can be overcome when the clinical social worker speaks the same language and is aware of the clients/patient's ethnicity. Lumb, D. (1999), defined cultural competence as "the group of knowledge and skills that social workers and other health care professionals have in order to be competent with multicultural patients." Multicultural social work deals with different components of culture which includes, race, gender, age, sexual orientation, religion. Green, J. (1982-1999), author of "Cultural awareness in the Human Services" was aware when he said that the practice of ethnically competency requires knowledge base, professional training, and adequate interventions to be able to compare and understand diverse cultures. Culture is a group of learning beliefs, shared values, styles of communication, practice, costumes, and points of view about roles and relationships (Betancourt, J.R., 2004).

The daily activities of the author with Spanish speaking clients/patients, provide an understanding about the complexity of bilingual and cultural communication in the hospital setting and community mental health settings. These experiences can also be extended to other clients/patients of other foreign languages. Those clinical social workers who do not speak the language of clients/patients often find themselves experiencing communication problems.

Cultural competence obstacles:

Even though language is important, this is not the only obstacle. Obstacles can be any aspect of attention of health care that contributes to the wrong use of it. Obstacles can affect the quality of services that are offered and may also contribute to racial and ethnic disparities, which include:

1. Lack of diversity in health care centers.
2. The health care center is inadequately designed to fulfil the needs of a diverse population of clients/patients.
3. Communication problems among health care providers and clients/patients of different ethnic groups, culture, language, social and religions.

Cultural competence is one of the principal ingredients for the elimination of disparities in community health care centers, and for that reason when clinical social workers speak of psychosocial and mental health problems without understanding cultural differences that are brought during the interaction with the clients/patients, these can be intensified. Simply said, those community mental health centers that respect and respond to the sociocultural and linguistics of a diverse population, can help for the creation of positive results of mental health care services. For the development of cultural competence, is needed to examine preferences and prejudices, searching for models to follow and to share as much as possible with other people who have the passion for cultural competence. The term multicultural competence came from the publication in Mental health by the psychologist Paul Pedersen in 1998, at competency requires least a decade before the term cultural competence became popular.

Without cultural awareness, social workers contribute to oppression when working with clients/patients from other cultures. This is unethical practice and can cause clients/patients great harm (Sue, D., Arredonde, P., McDavis, R., 1992). Clinical social workers need skills to assess client/patients' entire system. If ignored, they may echo society's oppression by assuming that clients/patients need to change, rather than working for societal change (Pinderhughes, E., 1989). Also, cultural competence can also lead to overcompensation by clinical social workers and may spend unnecessary time focusing on culture or may excuse dysfunctional behavior (Comas-Diaz, L., 1995).

According to Coon, D. (2000), most definitions of cultural competence are shared with a diversity of professionals that are from the mental health field. According to Carter, R. (1999), some of the benefits of developing cultural competence in any organization, are:

1. Increases respect and mutual understanding among those involved.
2. Increases creativity to solve problems through new perspectives, ideas, and strategies.
3. Decreases unwanted surprises that could delay progress in the intervention.
4. Increases trust and cooperation from the client/patient.
5. Increases participation and collaboration with other multicultural groups.
6. Helps to overcome fear of making mistakes, to competence or conflict. For example, by understanding and accepting people from diverse cultures, there are more probabilities that these people will feel comfortable.
7. Promote the inclusion and equality of rights.

Statistical data of Latinos in the United States:

In 2005, the Latino population was the largest minority group in the United States, consisting of: 14% of the total population, compared with 13% of African Americans and 5% of Asians. For next 2059, it is expected that the Latinos will be 29% of the population. According to the US Census Bureau (2006) and the Pew Hispanic Center (2015), more than double the representation for 2005. New York State is the home of more than 3.1 million Latinos or 16% of the population (Pew Hispanic Center, 2015). Latinos of Caribbean descendants are the largest group of people from Latin America (58%), followed by those of Latin American descendants (15%), follow by (12%) of Mexican descendants and (9%) of Central America.

According to the Pew Hispanic Center report (2015), Latinos are 25% of the total population of New York State; 38% are White, 23% are African Americans and 14% are from Asia and the Pacific Islands. Most Latinos live in East Harlem, New York, in "El Barrio" as it is referred by the Latino residents. According to the 2000 US Census, Latinos were 52.1% of the population of East Harlem, New York, followed by 35% African Americans, Whites 7.7%. Among Latinos, Puerto Ricans are the largest group in East Harlem or 57.75% of the population, followed by 16.9% of Mexicans, and 7.7% from the Dominican Republic. According to the Pew Hispanic Center (2015), the Latino population has grown 14% or 2'485,260. According to the New York Controller's Office (2016), almost one in every New Yorker defines themselves as Latino or Hispanic. Between 1990 and 2014, the Latino population in New York State has increased 66%, reaching 3.7 million (19%) of the population, and most of them live in the New York City Metropolitan area.

The Latino contribution to the United States:

According to the US Census Bureau (2016), in the State of New York, 83% of Latinos do not speak English in their homes. Lack of English ability is a major obstacle for their access to medical and mental health services. Most importantly yet, those who preferred to get mental health services in Spanish had less probabilities of access to mental health services. Compared with those Latinos with English ability, those with limited knowledge of English were 65 years old or older, with higher probabilities for having medical insurance. All these factors contribute to the risk of emotional stress.

According to the US Census Bureau (2016), of the 50 million of Latinos who make the most contribution to the demographic development in the United States and who continue to be in vast majority, are Mexicans, Puerto Ricans, and Cubans. The face of most of this country is changing. The numbers of the 2010 US Census prove that Latinos are more than 16% of the population and their number is growing to a 43% in the last decade. Latinos contributed between 2000 and 2010 to the 56% of the increased of the total population of this country. The financial recession hit Latinos especially hard with the construction crisis, an important sector of employment for this minority group and only in 2009, 1,4 million Latinos were added to this group of poor people that in the United States is decided by an annual salary well below $22,000.

According to the US Census Bureau (2016), the poverty rate among Latinos was 23.4% compared to White people or 12.4%, Afro-Americans 26.2%, Native Americans 27.6%, meanwhile Asians were 12.3%. The level of education of Latinos is notably inferior to the general population, 23.5% of Latinos have completed less of nine years of high school compared to 6.3% of the general population, 3% of White and 5.4% of African Americans. The other extreme of academic education, only 12% of Latinos have graduated from a university, compared to the general population, 31.1% of Whites and 17%.7% of African Americans. Although the rhythm of growth of the Latino population has decreased in recent years, the office of Census calculates that for the year 2050 there will be about one hundred million Latinos. This is 25% of the general population.

What is considered good health for Latinos?

According to a survey conducted with doctors and Latino patients in New York City, there is a vast disparity among Latino patients and their doctors about what they think about having good health. While many Latinos think that their health is good, their doctors disagreed in large numbers (Tallaj, R., M., 2018). And only one third of Latinos think that they do not get the medical attention they need, while two thirds of the doctors think that Latinos have persistent barriers to have access to medical and mental health services. Most medical and mental health problems are left unattended within the Latino community. Smoking, asthma, obesity, diabetes, arterial hypertension, and anxiety are some of the main health problems, but education in this area is comparable with the seriousness of this issue, and reports about health education are not available in Spanish (Tallaj, R., 2018).

The level of education of Latinos is inferior to that of general population. Among the adult Latinos in New York City, between the ages of 25 and more, 35% did not graduated from high school, compared to the 14% among adult Latinos. A lower percentage of Latinos compared with non-Latinos have completed college, 16% vs. 42% (US Bureau of Census, 2018). Although the growth rhythm of the Latino population has recently decreased, the US Bureau of Census (2018), estimates that by next 2030 there will be 74.81 million of Latinos in the United States.

The US Bureau of Census (2018) expects the adult Latino population to grow about 55% in the next three decades, compared with the rest of the White population. The adult Latino population has more probabilities of being poor. 24% of adult Latinos (compared with 12% of Whites). Poor health condition appears to attribute to the low financial level and the time exposed to occupations that affect their health (construction, landscaping, carpentry, agriculture, etc.). Putting them together, the access to healthcare services for this population is extremely limited (NKI center for excellence in Culturally Competent Mental Health, 2011).

Every year, mental health problems affect millions of Americans and Latinos are not an exception. The immigrant Latino population and their children find an alarming number of risk factors and emotional problems. Also, their limited minority condition and citizenship could limit their access to services that they need. According to a report from Zárate, M. (2003) while the mental health problems are the result of a combination of genes and environmental factors. Environmental circumstances also play a key role.

Children of immigrants may have difficulty living with expectations and demands of a culture in their home and another in school. The children may not go to their parents whenever they have problems or worries, thinking that their parents do not understand the culture enough to be able to help them or that they be too stressed with other stressors due to their settlement. While the second and third generation of immigrants faces higher risks of emotional problems, many Latino immigrants do not receive mental health treatment only when their condition is terrible. The Latino immigrants are underrepresented in the healthcare and mental health care system, and in treatment of problems that not needed hospitalization (NKI Center for Excellence in Culturally Competent Mental Health, 2011). This means that often doctor's offices do not take care of persons with emotional problems or could have the risk of hurting themselves or others. It is not fair that when a person enters a doctor's office suffering from an emotional problem (anxiety/depression), and the first question is *"do you have medical insurance" did you bring your insurance card"*?

Latinos have the highest rate of not having medical insurance among any other group in the United States. Lack of medical insurance prevents the access to medical and mental health services. In 2007, 32% of the Latino population did not have medical insurance compared to the White non-Latino population, 10.4% (Pew Research Center, 2009). The index is higher for older Mexican Americans, 37.6% than Puerto Ricans, 20.4%, and Cubans, 22% of younger than 65 do not have medical insurance. Children make 29% of younger than 19 and 8 years old who do not have medical insurance, compared with 11% of Whites of the same age (NKI Center of Excellence in Culturally Competent Mental Health, 2011). The reason for the lack of medical insurance, according to the US Bureau of Census (2018), is because employers do not offer medical insurance and only 44% of Latinos who have medical insurance it is due to citizenship, level of education and characteristics of place of employment.

Latinos' needs and demands for mental health services will increase as the population grows. Without efforts to understand how Latinos cope with mental health problems, what factors influence access to mental health services, and how to deliver quality mental health services to them. Latinos will continue to suffer disproportionally from unmet mental health needs (Vega, WA., Lopez, S.R., 2001). Latino adults in need of mental health care are less likely than non-Latino white to access mental health services, and when they do receive care, it is more likely to be poor in quality (Institute of Medicine (IOMD), 2003; United States Department of Health and Human Services (USDHHS), 2001

The level of acculturation among Latinos in the United States may be a factor to predict emotional problems and the evidence of the role of acculturation has been consistent. (Ortega,

A. N., 2000), reported the possibility of increased emotional problems and alcohol abuse and substance abuse among Latinos acculturated than non-acculturated to the United States. The way of living in the United States imposes cultural changes and stress in the way Latinos used to live in their county. Adapting to the American culture could weaken the family structure (familism), is there is not a solid family system and the mental health of parents, and their children could worsen (Comas-Diaz, L., Niño, M., 2019). According to these authors, Latino immigrants have better health and mental health than Latinos who were born in the United States.

The strong family orientation, also known as familism, could contribute to their immigrant advantage. Because of the increasing monolingual and bilinguals among the Latino population in the United States, it is important for clinical social workers to be culturally competent and sensitive to be able to obtain positive results. It is this author's opinion that when services are offered in the language of the client/patient without need of a translator, Latinos continue the treatment longer than when the services are not provided in their own language.

Family, its importance, and its main socioeconomic transformations:

In the United States, immigrant families must avoid many challenges related to economic condition, health care, housing, and education for their children. Some obstacles are lack of education, not being able to read or speak English, lack of familiarity with American's way of life, difficulty to find stable employment, or one that pays enough to be able to support the family and the difficulty of having access to welfare aid, health, and mental health services.

When we talk about Latino family immigrants, the father is the role model who transmits example, and values to his children. His absence is detrimental for the family. Simply he is not there in his house, his home, with his children, with his family because he is out working long hours of the day. And unfortunately, because of the many reasons families break up, even though they have links that united them, there is migration. Migration is the process of separation that is more difficult, because the family members have not broken their emotional links, but these are broken by the distance, even if is for a better life. But *what does it mean a better life when we must be apart from our loved ones? Why many times we only talk about the immigrant suffering separating from his family, but what about the suffering of his parents, his wife, his children, the girlfriend, the fiancée, his friends, his siblings, spaces, their costumes, the neighborhood, a life, the counterpart, the suffering of the family when they see their son, friend go away?* Because of varied reasons, aimlessly, with only a goal of a dream which is what keeps steady in his decision to leave, with the disappointment of his country or his city, with many injustices, with his family in his heart and mind, there is no fear, at least it should not be mentioned because it weakens him/her.

Advice for more mental health services:

The increase of mental health problems in the Latino community, in New York City, is alarming. It has been worsened by current health care problems like Covid-19 (coronavirus). It is also alarming for Latin America, where the resources are scarce. For this reason, clinical social work in mental health should be expanded, with emphasis on education, promotion, and prevention of mental health problems. Clinical social workers provide mental health services to individuals, groups and families who have emotional problems, through diagnosis and psychotherapy. It is also important to note that the actual family context is more complex, due to the way that marital relationships are formalized and ruptured.

The stress of acculturation is particularly difficult for Latino families with parents who are monolingual and with their children who are bilingual and have problems adapting to the American culture. According to a report from the American Psychological Association (2013), titled, "The Psychology of Immigration in the New Century," parents of immigrant Latinos and their children live in different worlds and often parents do not know much of what their children do when they are out of their home. This situation puts pressure on their children to look for an exit to their problems and what advice their parents can give to them. Even though there is an increase of need for professional servicers among Latino families and access to professional mental health services, many families do not seek these services due to the stigma that surrounds mental health.

The American Psychological Association (2013), recommends that mental health services should be developed in three phases:

1. Cultural knowledge of the psychotherapist.
2. Attitudes and beliefs of the psychotherapist towards the different attitudes of clients/patients.
3. Beliefs of clients/patients and personal understanding, skills of the psychotherapist and adequate therapeutic interventions available. This includes offering to clients/patients, easy access to resources such as, translators and legal aide, as well as easing access to different community programs available in the community.

Also necessary is the interdisciplinary intervention among agencies of the health care system. It is this author's opinion that there should be a transition of collaboration of services without interruptions among hospitals, schools, and community mental health centers. By doing so, patients will continue receiving mental health services without delays. The mental health system can also help to improve the mental health of the Latino communities by finding them where they are. There should be information campaigns along with media networks in different languages, in places where the Latino immigrant gather such as, churches, social clubs (American Psychological Association, 2013).

Interdisciplinary clinical social work:

According to Abramson, J., & Mizrahi, T. (1996), Garcés, C., 2018-2019), the reasoning for participation and collaboration among health care professionals is based on the recognition of the complexity of human problems, level of knowledge and intervention that is necessary to obtain positive results. The clinical social worker intensifies the effectiveness of his intervention that is necessary to get positive results. The clinical social worker intensifies the effectiveness of his intervention by having knowledge of the culture and history of a client/patient. Culture and traditions are important components. It is also important for the client/patient and his/her family to be able to share his/her traditions with the clinical social worker during the first interview. A good personal question could be: *What is important in your culture that would help me to be able to offer my services?* The answer to this question could help to prevent misunderstandings between the clinical social worker and the client/patient and family members (Garcés, C., 2018- 2919).

Common mental health problems among the Latino community in New York:

Latinos have the same incidence of mental health problems when compared to the rest of the New York population. However, certain concerns, experiences, ways of understanding them and how to manage them could be different. Without mental health we cannot be healthy. Any part of the human body, including the brain, could get sick. We all go through different events or situations that occasionally can cause emotional difficulties. Mental health problems go beyond our emotional reactions that we go through during different situations. It has to do with some situations or conditions that could change our routine, because these can get complicated and could also create relationship problems with other people, as well as in the work setting and lose employment. Without adequate treatment, mental health problems could get worse and make the daily life of a person difficult (National Alliance on Mental Illness, 2019).

Symptoms of mental health problems:

1. Trouble concentrating, remembering details, and making decisions.
2. Fatigue.
3. Feeling guilt, worthlessness, and helplessness.
4. Pessimism and hopelessness.
5. Insomnia, early-morning wakefulness, or sleeping too much.
6. Crankiness or irritability.
7. Restlessness.
8. Loss of interest in things once pleasurable, including sex.
9. Overeating, or appetite loss.
10. Aches, pains, headaches, or cramps that don't get better, even with treatment.
11. Digestive problems that don't get better, even with treatment.
12. Persistent sad, anxious, or "empty" feelings.
13. Suicidal thoughts.

The most common mental health problems in the Latino community:

1. Schizophrenia
2. General anxiety disorder
3. Major depression
4. Stress disorder
5. Bipolar disorder

Other problems associated within mental health with the Latino community:

1. Suicidal attempts
2. Excessive use of illicit drugs and alcohol

Domestic violence

Nonetheless, the Latino community in New York shows a similar predisposition to the mental health conditions when compared to the rest of the population. Sadly, there are many inequalities to mental health and quality of treatment. This inequality exposes a considerable risk for Latinos of having a mental health breakdown or crisis situations and be able to be treated adequately. Generally, Latinos do not seek mental health treatment. According to the Administration of Substance and Mental Health, in 2012, only 27% of Latinos with mental health related problems sought professional help. The people in the Latino communities' do not talk about their mental health problems. There is not enough information on this issue, and we cannot know what has not been taught us. Many Latinos do not seek mental health treatments because they do not recognize the symptoms or because they do not know where to get help. This lack of information worsens the stigma already associated with mental health problems. Also, Latinos do not seek mental health treatment out fear of being labeled as "crazy," since this could cause them shame.

The stress of acculturation according to Dillon, F., & et.al, (2013), has to do with the psychological stress that is experienced by immigrants when responding to the challenges they meet while adjusting to a different culture. Decades of research studies has sparked interest about the impact of mental health problems among Latinos in the United States, making this a frequent determinant of inequalities in mental health services for Latinos. Acculturative stress is linked to multiple psychosocial and mental health problems, including, anxiety, depression, suicide, alcohol, and illegal drug abuse. Despite this, there is not enough understanding about the experiences that are related to acculturative stress during the first years of immigrating to the United States.

Latinos in New York face factors that could increase their risk of mental health problems. Stress could manifest itself through depression and anxiety, which could lead to the use and abuse of illegal drugs and alcohol, and in some instances, in suicide. Stress is also manifested through immigration, which is the cause of emotional distress, and to many immigrants the transition of relocation is problematic. According to Insel, T. R. (2005), the systemic investigation within the moratorium trajectory and the later follow up of the cultural, social, vocational indicators of the family functioning could help clinical social workers to recognize problems, adjustments and to engage in the promotion of mental health, prevention, and treatment interventions in each time. Due to the limited evidence of studies, more research would help to evaluate intervention strategies for the promotion of mental health in the Latino communities for the prevention of mental health problems that respond to problems of acculturation.

Cultural differences could be the cause for clinical social workers to incorrectly diagnose their clients/patients. For example, Latinos usually describe their symptoms that are related to depression with "nervousness, fatigue, or physically ill." These symptoms are related to depression. However, when the clinical social worker does not understand the client's/patient's culture, this too could influence the treatment negatively, and not be able to recognize the symptoms of depression with "nervousness, fatigue, or physically ill." These symptoms are related to depression. However, when the clinical social worker does not understand the client's/patient's culture, this too may influence the treatment negatively, and may hinder recognizing symptoms of depression.

Both the presentation of emotional problems and the way they are explained by Latinos in the United States are different. According to Lewis-Fernandez, E, et al. (2005), Latinos with depression problems have more probability of presenting themselves with psychosomatic complaints when compared with White Americans. This may be the reason that Latinos are more apt to seek medical treatment for these problems instead of seeking mental health treatment. It is important that the somatic presentation of depression among Latinos may cause doctors to make mistakes, ending up with a wrong diagnosis, unnecessary medical exams, and inadequate treatment (Lewis-Fernandez, et al., 2005).

Latinos have diverse ways in defining their emotional problems. Some Latinos believe in spirits or sins for the cause of their illness; an interpretation that to this date has not been understood by mental health care professionals. They may use different language that prevents recognition and understanding of their problems. Lack of success in distinguishing common emotional cultural problems may contribute to the delay in seeking help, inadequate treatment, and negative results.

A known cultural disorder among Latinos is *"nervous attack,"* "which is a language of desperation. It is particularly common among Latinos from the Caribbean and is well recognized by many Latinos. This is described in the Diagnostic Criteria of the DSM-5 (2013) of cultural disorders and the symptoms include: Uncontrolled chills, crying attacks, body shakes, heat in the chest area to the head, turning verbally or physically aggressive. Typically, nervous attack occurs because of a stress event, especially related to family problems. Frequently, after the nervous attack it is common for the person to suffer amnesia of what has taken place, but soon after returns to his/her normal functioning. Frequently, the nervous attack is compared with an episode of panic attack due to the similarity of the symptoms. Both, panic attacks and nervous attacks have a closed association with the absence of symptoms of fear and panic (Guarmaccia, P.J., 2008). Because nervous attack is described as a temporary emotional reaction to circumstances of daily life, the person may not recognize the debilitating emotional problem or the need to seek professional mental health services (NKI Center for Excellence in Culturally Competent Mental Health, 2009).

While the fear symptoms are like the ones in the DSM-5 Diagnostic and Statistical Criteria Manual of Mental Disorders (2013) of depression the complications for its treatment are different. Traditionally, the treatment for fear consists in a practice of cultural rituals, with the purpose of calling the soul to come back to the body to "clean" the affected person and return the total balance to his/her body. Such rituals are known by the traditional Latin traditional healer. While those clients/patients who suffer from scare can experience some improvement in the conventional treatment for symptoms of major depression, lack of consideration of the cultural believes of clients/patients may limit the efficiency of the therapeutic intervention, affect the adherence, and change the trust (or lack of trust) in the sector of formal mental health. The event the precipitates fear could be correlative with the western differential diagnosis. For example, fear because of a conflict of a major correlation with the western differential diagnosis of major depression disorder (Guarmaccia, P. J., 2008).

The challenges are even greater for people who only speak Spanish and have to go to an interview with a clinical social worker who does not speak their language to talk about their problems. Translation can be helpful, but the clinical social worker should have a good understanding of the cultural context to be able to help the client/patient. Different dialects may also complicate the translation. Many Latino immigrants do not seek professional mental health help or trust clinical social workers due to the lack of cultural understanding and the professional competency to understand their problems. According to The National Alliance on Mental health (2017), one of each five Latinos suffers from a mental health problem. Latinos have a collective orientation, being family orientation (familism), of mutual help and united, this are family ties of the Latino culture (National Alliance on Mental Health, 2011). Familism, a unique word in the Spanish language that emphasizes a strong family relationship, may help as a protective factor that promotes social support which protects people against symptoms of depression, including considerable risk of environmental situations (National Alliance on Mental Health, 2011).

Even though major depression in the Latin woman is being recognized, the risk and the mechanisms of protection that are associated with the effects in children when the mother suffers from depression, is well understood by Latino families. During the 2000 census, Latino women were 51% of the Latino population in the United States (Bureau of Census, 2000). Most Latino women are concentrated in occupations of low salaries. They work in factories, restaurants, house cleaning, hair salons, receptionists, laundry shops, flower shops. The Latino women have double unemployment when compared with Caucasian American women and suffer multiple social and economic disadvantages such as low level of education, unemployment, low income, single mothers, elevated levels of poverty and victims of domestic violence. These factors affect their mental health and limit their access to health and mental health care services. Latino women who are born in the United States have a higher risk level of major depression and suicide attempts than non-Latino women (Giachello, A., 2001).

A study by Lewis, M. J., et al. (2005), found significant levels of stigma associated to symptoms of depression and antidepressant medication. Latinos who took part in the study and received treatment for depression said that an experience with depressive symptoms is described negatively, seen as a characteristic within the social context. When the same people were interviewed about the complications adhering to antidepressant medication therapy, 73% of participants made comments with reference to stigma, antidepressant medication, followed by 87% of side effects from the medication. Having to take antidepressant medication appears to be disapproved by families of the participants and of their social system support. Family members may also discourage their loved ones from seeking treatment or taking medications due to a lack of education or spiritual or cultural beliefs.

Even though Latinos prefer to be treated by Latino mental health professionals, unfortunately this is not possible due to the small percentage of Latino clinical social workers or bilingual clinical social workers who are culturally competent. To understand the reasons for cultural disparities, it will help us to build a mental health system that can be able to combine the superior quality of effective mental health services. Latinos conform one third of the eight million habitants of New York City. But even when Latinos are a substantial part of the state of New York, and no sooner are an increasing population, they keep themselves invisible. Latinos are invisible because they are different, and with these factors together, the attention of their health and mental health is in crisis. Compared with New York residents, Latino immigrants lack health care benefits and lack quality medical care. Latino immigrants face that makes them more at risk of getting sick (Tallaj, R.M 2018).

Immigration and acculturation may be stressful and even traumatizing for some people. Immigration often separates families from their extended family, resulting in an enormous loss of support (Heyck, D., 1994). U.S. immigration policies and practices may be intimidating, unwelcoming, and even violent (Gutierrez, L., Yeakley., Ortega, R. 2000); this may lead to a generalized fear or distrust for social services.

Mental health services vs. home remedy (Botanical)

The low index of using mental health services among the Latino population is attributed to the social consequences of seeking these services. The study suggests that Latinos do not seek help due of fear of deportation, mistrust of providers and fear to authorities (Lewis, M. J., et al., 2005). Other studies suggest that people are afraid to bring shame to the family when seeking mental health services. According to the same study Latinos see emotional problems as something very private and it should not be shared with others outside the family. Latinos may be less ready and fit than White Americans in seeking mental health services because their mental health is supported by the family. Social resources include family, friends, godparents, religious affiliations, spiritual and other people that practice healings and groups of personal help. These resources are often used instead of professional mental health services. However, literature suggests that these resources do not effectively replace professional services.

Stigma about mental health among Latinos in New York:

According to the World Health Organization (2016), mental health stigma is the largest community barrier to improving global mental health, and in Latin American cultures, this stigma may be more prevalent. The WHO reports that stigma surrounding mental ill-health is the biggest obstacle in the way of people seeking treatment. Stigma refers to a set of negative, and often unfair or inaccurate, beliefs that society associates with certain circumstances, qualities, or people. Mental health stigma refers to negative attitudes or beliefs that lead to the devaluating, disgracing, and disfavoring by of individuals with mental illness. There are three commonly recognized types of mental health stigma (Mascayo, F., Tapia, T., et al., 2016):

1. **Social or public stigma:** This refers to the negative discriminatory beliefs or attitudes about mental health conditions promoted in one's cultural group or broader society.
2. **Self-stigma:** This occurs when a person internalizes negative societal attitudes about mental health conditions.
3. **Institutional stigma:** This refers to government or private institutional policies that intentionally or intentionally discriminate against people with mental health conditions.

Mental health stigma is still a major negative influencing factor in how people both treat and perceive mental health conditions. Mental health stigma exists everywhere in the world, but it may be particularly strong in Latin American cultures and communities (Mascayo, F.; Tapia, T., et al. (2016).

Commonly identified stigmas that people with mental health problems are:

1. Violent, aggressive, or likely to act out of the ordinary.
2. Incapable of getting better.
3. Dangerous and should be isolated or kept away from the public.
4. Cannot perform the same activities or duties as others.

Some elements of Latin American culture that may influence how mental health stigma is set, perceived, and affected:

1. Familism:

The cultural value of familism, or the collective value of family unity, can play a role in shaping and enforcing mental health stigma among Latinos (National Alliance on Mental health, 2011). This value can be associated with increased rates of hostile attitudes from family and extended family, as well as family members underestimating someone's abilities. Upon learning the psychiatric diagnosis, families often experienced frustration, denial, and grief (Uribe, R., et al., 2007). Discussing mental health problems is often a taboo. This means that they avoid talking about this topic among family members and friends.

2. Religion:

Religious worship and church activities are part of Latino cultural socialization. Spirituality is important for Latinos and is a source of emotional support (Gelman, C., 2004). While most Latinos are Catholic, one should not assume all families are Catholic or particularly devout. Some Latinos believe in spirits and folk healing, termed "curanderismo." Latino clients/patients may also seek healing through folk medicine while receiving professional health/mental health care (Comas-Diaz, L, 1995).

Faith also plays a role in shaping the stigma that Latinos may hold about mental health problems. Latinos tend to rely on religious institutions as an important spiritual, educational, and social resource. According to a 2019 study exploring beliefs about mental health conditions in faith-based Latin communities in New York. Religious beliefs may contribute to stigmas by enforcing the misconceptions that:

1. Mental ill-health is a moral failing or spiritual dilemma.
2. Mental ill-health is a spiritual, rather than a medical, condition.
3. Mental ill-health is a punishment or form of divine justice.
4. Depression Is due to a lack of faith, not praying enough, sinful behaviors towards parents or others, or demonic influence. Praying and having faith in God can help reduce the risk of or treat mental health conditions.
5. Lack of true faith.

Latinos living in the New York may also have reduced access to proper mental health care due to the following factors:

1. Language barriers.
2. Lack of healthcare providers aware of Latin American cultural differences, beliefs, language nuances, or practices.
3. Lack of specialized healthcare resources in the community.
4. A reduced ability to find the symptoms of mental ill-health due to a lack of information or understanding.
5. Legal status or status of a loved one.
6. How much someone adjusts and accepts the predominant culture of where they are living.
7. Poverty.
8. How much someone adjusts and accepts the predominant culture of where they were living.

To **reduce the stigma surrounding mental ill-health, the National Alliance on Mental Illness (2011), recommended the following:**

1. Talking openly about mental health.
2. Educating oneself and others about mental health.
3. Promoting the idea that physical and mental ill-health are the same.
4. Being aware of language that may be stigmatizing, such as the terms "crazy," "insane," or "psychotic."
5. Letting media outlets know when they are promoting negative stigma.
6. Showing compassion to people with mental health conditions.

Botanicals (ethnic stores of home remedies) are particularly found in New York City. Botanicals are stores that offer religious home remedies, spiritual products and services to a diverse client which are mostly from Latin America and the Caribbean countries. The presence of botanicals in New York City is related to the presence of dispensaries (drugstores that appeared in 1900). These botanicals are in areas where Latinos are the majority. Also, the botanicals offer counseling services to people who look for spiritual and emotional guidance in a variety of situations, from financial to emotional problems (counseling). The belief of the effectiveness of home practice, combined with medicinal herbs that offered in the botanicals are cheap (low cost), and of easy access, bring Latinos who seek informal mental health services (Gómez, A., Beloz, J., et al (2011).

In a recent study by Perez Porto, M. (2017-2019), traditional healers are said to be able to cure a wide variety of physiological, spiritual, and emotional sufferings. They are also said to have a unique way to diagnose and to cure, compared to the model of the United States: psychosomatic causes which are the result of social demand. Latinos with physical and emotional problems have the tendency to make less use of mental health services than White Americans. In 2007, only 26.6%

of Latinos with serious mental health problems received services, compared with 50% of White Latinos.

Professional personal use:

The practice of clinical social work with Latinos demands a careful personal evaluation and understanding of how social workers see the world around them and how the dominant society affects their professional intervention with Latinos. Therefore, social workers need to be aware of their own bias and how their world view affects their concept of clients/patients. For example, if a social worker's point of view is to value individualism, he/she should critically assess how to address a client/patient from a collective point of view (Furman, R., and colleagues., 2006).

Latinos value intimate personal relationships. They also value the role of the clinician and tend to adopt a "doctor/patient" tradition, specially at the beginning of the professional relationship. It is also important to understand why Latinos would like to know the personal life of the clinician. They tend to question about family and friends of the clinician. Clinical social workers must understand that this is not a matter of professional boundaries but part of the culture. Non-Latino clinical social workers must be sensitive to this and may need to adapt their style to the expectations of Latino clients/patients. Some modifications may include an increased amount of self-disclosure, accepting gifts (often food), and more physical contact (handshakes, pats on the back), as well as being closer spatially (Gelman, C., 2004). Nonverbal behavior and time awareness are also important traits. Many Latinos are comfortable with close interpersonal space (Gutierrez, L., Yeakley, A., Ortega, R., 2000). This may result in confusion about appointment time and scheduling. The clinical social worker's cultural awareness is critical to prevent misunderstanding (Gelman, C., 2004).

Social workers in mental health:

Because of the exeunt of social workers in hospitals, social workers had to find new roles for themselves. They decided to enter areas of mental health and make themselves useful in this regard. This promotion in mental health has a history (National Institute of Mental Health, 1991). From psychiatry hospitals to the development of community mental health centers, social workers have found themselves providing psychotherapy to individuals, groups, and families. Also, social workers have been active in the actual prevention of mental illness caused by current world events like Covid-19. They have made efforts to develop public programs and distribute funds, to make sure that mental illness is treated with the same degree of gravity as other medical illnesses.

By working with other mental health professionals (psychologists, psychiatrists), clinical social workers began to collaborate in the development of theories of ethology and interventions, which have been now tried through practice and research. However, unbeknown to be unsuspecting investigator, emphasis on mental health instead of the social environment has changed the historical course of the typical social worker. Instead of the individual and his environment, the clinical social worker looks to justify practice on the same grounds as the medical doctor or nurse, who subscribes to the bio-psychosocial approach to the consumer. This may seem like a small detail in a large panoramic view of the place of the clinical social worker in society, but it is not a small gnat or fly in the ointment. Presently, clinical social workers work on the psyche of the individual, helping his/her to find happiness, peace inside of him/herself and to better their mental health. The consumer's social environment has fallen by the historical wayside. The main goal of clinical social workers in mental health is to be able to help people who suffer from mental illness, so that they can function in the world in which they live. This new adopted role has helped to improve the conditions for the mentally ill, who are no longer locked up in psychiatric institutions. The concept subscribed to now by the clinical social worker helps the consumer "adjust" to the realities of life (National Institute of Mental Health, 1991).

Unlike the psychiatrists and psychologists, clinical social workers are trained to have interest in the whole person. Yet, these new adopted roles and environments are challenging, for the medical model is hard to squash. It prevails, and this means that the clinical social worker's training to treat the whole person bumps head-on into psychiatry's focus, which is to cure the illness by prescribing psychotropic medication (National Institute of Mental Health, 1991). What this really means is even the adopted role of the clinical social worker, to be the advocate for the mentally ill, has also been challenged as well. The typical clinical social worker in a psychiatric hospital or a community mental health clinic has his/her hands tied to the psychiatrist who may not really believe that psychotherapy conducted by a clinical social worker helps the patient as much as an anti-psychotic medication. If this is true, it might have been wiser for the clinical social worker to remain in the hospital setting, where becoming an orphan to be adopted was not an option.

This author's professional experience in community mental health began after graduating from Fordham University in 1985. It was in the Puerto Rican family Institute in the South Bronx, New York where he first worked as a psychiatric social worker. The people in the South Bronx were mainly Puerto Ricans, from the Dominican Republic and from other countries of Latin America. Later, in 1997 he went to work Queens Neuropsychiatric Institute in Jackson Heights Queens, New York where most of the clients/patients are from Perú, Chile, Argentina, Ecuador, Bolivia, México, Colombia, Uruguay, Venezuela. Since 2010 he has been working as a psychotherapist at Community Counseling Services on Long Island, New York where the clients/patients are mixed; Americans and Latinos, mostly from Honduras, El Salvador, Guatemala, and México.

According to a report from the World Health Organization (WHO-2013), mental health is defined as a state of wellbeing in which an individual is aware of his/her own capabilities, is capable to face normal life's stressors, can work productively and capable to contribute to the community. The positive dimension of mental health stands out in the definition of health listed in the Constitution of the World Health Organization (2013): Health is a state of complete physical, mental, and social wellbeing, and not only about the absence of affections or illness. Mental health includes our emotional, psychological, and social wellbeing. It affects the way we think, feel, and behave when facing challenging problems. It also helps to decide how we manage emotional stress, how we relate with other people and how we make decisions. Mental health is important in all phases of our life from birth to the end of life.

Understanding clinical social work:

Clinical social work is a type of specialty of medical social work which deals with counseling, psychotherapy, and coordinating services (discharge planning) to individuals with severe mental health problems, and in certain situations need psychiatric hospitalization or other psychiatric treatment. Clinical social workers have a variety of tasks when treating clients/patients, including but not limited to psychosocial evaluations, individual, family and group psychotherapy, crisis intervention, emotional support, and coordinating medical attention and discharge planning. Clinical social workers are employed in a variety of settings: Hospitals, court system, schools, drug and rehabilitation centers, nursing and rehabilitation centers, community mental health centers.

Clinical social work is a specialty that meets the following requirements:

1. Has a systemic body of theories that supports what it does.
2. Has professional authority emanating from the domain of theory.
3. Has community knowledge that the profession is valid.
4. Has a code of ethics that governs the conduct of its members, has a professional culture within a vocabulary, and professional method.

Clinical social work bases its method in the systemic field of evidence based in knowledge derived from research and practical evaluation, including its own knowledge and a specific content. It also acknowledges the complex interactions among people and their environment, and the ability of individuals to react when they are affected by multiple influences or circumstances upon themselves, including psychosocial, health and environmental factors such as the COVID-19. The social work profession extracts from theories of human development, social theory, and social systems theory to analyze complex situations, and familiarize individual changes of cultural and social organizations (NASW Definition of Social Work, 2000).

Clinical social workers provide mental health services (psychotherapy) to individuals, families, and groups of individuals who have emotional problems. Clinical social workers provide psychotherapy and diagnose emotional problems by using the DSM-5 Diagnostic and Statistical Manual of Mental Disorders (2013). The role of the clinical social worker varies according of the setting of practice. In the hospital setting is mostly discharge planning. This starts as soon as the patient is admitted to the hospital and takes place upon the patient's discharge from the hospital. Sometimes patients need special services such as, referrals to nursing and rehabilitation nursing homes, orthopedic rehabilitation, drug, and alcohol rehabilitation (Garcés, C., 2018-2019). During the discharge planning, the clinical social worker must make sure that the patient has all the necessary resources before going back home and to be able to function in the community. Presently, hospital stay is shorter than a few years ago (Garcés, C., 2018-2019., NASW, 2007).

Psychiatric social work:

Psychiatric social work started simultaneously in John Hopkins Hospital in Boston. Garnet Pelton was the first social worker in 1907 and was assigned to the hospital's dispensary, known as Community Mental Health Center. Two years later Margaret Brogen, a nurse assumed the position and worked alone for several years. It became obvious to the hospital's administrators that her services were priceless, and the hospital would benefit by having more social workers to take care of patients. The Department of Social Work of the hospital became a formal part of the hospital in 1912, after the hospital started to hire more social workers. At that time social work education was in its first stages and most of the social workers were trained by nurses (NASW, 2007).

Psychiatric social work is a specialty of social work and follows the rehabilitation and restructuration of a patient's personality (takes place in psychiatric hospitals, community mental health centers, etc.), and psychosocial prophylaxis which deals with human mismatches. Psychiatric social work is the work of research about mental health problems, undertaking direct and responsible intervention along with psychiatry, with the aim to help patients who suffer from emotional problems. The psychiatric social worker is a professional who contributes to the prevention, treatment and rehabilitation of emotional problems working for it with the client/patient, his/her family with the goal to achieve social restoration.

The first psychiatric social workers with the support of Dr. Meyer from the Massachusetts General Hospital who, as well as Dr. Richard Cabot in 1905, understood that psychosocial factors have much to do with the genetics of emotional problems, and the social force could be introduced to improve their mental health. Dr. Meyer's wife, Mary Brooks Meyer, worked as a psychiatric social worker before she arrived at Baltimore. In her first position at the Pathologic Institute at New York Hospital in New York City, Ms. Meyer Brooks had already visited the homes of her patients and reported their conditions of their homes to her husband (NASW, 2007).

Psychiatric social workers work in psychiatric hospitals, community mental health clinics. Among other missions of psychiatric social work in the field of psychiatry there is:

1. The prevention of emotional problems through expected detection of susceptible cases.
2. The explanation to users of mental health services.
3. Implementation of measurements to improve follow up treatment such as, organizing family groups, self-help, collaboration in mental health awareness campaigns.

The clinical social worker:

Is a professional who is trained to evaluate and generate changes in the person who goes to his/her office for consultation and psychotherapy, which is given with the purpose to improve the quality of life through changes in the behavior and attitudes. The psychiatric social worker makes use of the FDS-5 Diagnostic and Statistical Manual of mental health (2013) for the evaluation of emotional problems. The psychiatric social worker is a licensed clinical social worker= who helps people to improve their lives, develop better cognitive and emotional skills, reduce symptoms of emotional distress to be able to face adversities. This professional is a person who helps people to remember that they are valued and appreciated by others too.

The clinical social worker as a family psychotherapist:

1. Educates family members about the role of the family as a group, particularly, how they function among themselves.
2. Helps the family to focus less on the member who was identified as "problematic," and to focused more on the family as a unit.
3. Helps to find conflicts and anxieties as well as to work together to develop strategies to solve them.
4. Strengthens all family members to be able to work together to solve problems.
5. Teaches ways to solve problems and changes within the family. Sometimes, the way that family members solve their problems makes them to have more probabilities to develop depressive symptoms.

Practice models of clinical social work (NASW, 2014):

1. **Resolution of problems.** The focus of this model is the understanding of the problem, searching for different ideas to solve the problem, allowing the client/patient to find a solution, to try the solution, and later, evaluate the outcome of the solution.
2. **Focus on homework.** The focus of this model is to separate the problem in small areas that the client/patient can achieve. The clinical social worker can use this as a practice, date limit and contract, to help the client/patient to be able to feel successful and motivated to solve the problem.
3. **Focus on the solution.** The focus of this model is to start with the solution, later to help the client/patient to stablish steps to arrive to the solution of the problem.
4. **Narrative.** The focus of this model is in using words and other models to help the client/patient to empower his/her life.
5. **Cognitive psychotherapy (CPT).** This model combines cognitive psychotherapy with behavioral psychotherapy, finding inadequate patterns of the thinking process, and
6. emotional answers, or behavior, substituting them with desirable patterns of thinking, emotional answers, or behavior. How to control anxiety and stress? Learning techniques of relaxation such as, deep breathing, talk aloud ana said: "I did this before," and distractions, finding situations that are often avoided, and gradually getting closer to fearful situations.

The difference between clinical social worker and clinical psychologist:

Frequently, clinical social workers and psychologists have the same functions. Clinical social workers can provide psychotherapy. Clinical social workers can address the mental, behavioral, or emotional health issues of clients/patients. Clinical social workers do not use psychological testing for diagnosis. Clinical social workers do not need a doctoral degree to practice.

Clinical psychologists study human behavior and can diagnose and treat mental illness, they use psychological testing for diagnosis. Both clinical social workers, and clinical psychologists have the goal of helping clients/patients with their problems through evaluation and treatment. Psychologists need a doctoral degree, while clinical social workers do not.

A clinical social worker Is the same as a counselor/psychologist?

When people talk about psychotherapy, they usually refer this term to psychotherapist, clinical social worker, psychologist, counselor within the context of collaborating with people to improve their mental health problems. These terms have the same meaning and can be interchanged. The use of the term over others is only about preference. Counselor and counseling are more common than psychotherapy and psychotherapist in the United States (NASW, 2014).

A list of different terms that Latinos in New York use as a synonymous of psychotherapy:

1. Counselor.
2. Mental health counselor.
3. Psychologist.

Psychotherapist, the meaning is the same, but people refer it to therapy. The term is useful because it can refer to a massage therapist, or another class of professional.

The attributes that are characteristic of clinical social work include the perspective of the use of respect by the person in the environment, for the importance of rights of clients/patients, and a strong therapeutic alliance between the client/patient and the clinical social worker. With more than 200,000 clinical social workers serving millions of clients/patients, clinical social workers are a large group of providers of mental health services in the United States (Center for Clinical Social Work, 2007-NASW, 2014).

The knowledge base of clinical social work includes theories of biology, psychological and sociological development, diversity and cultural competence, interpersonal relationships, family and group dynamics, mental health disorders, addictions, disease impact, traumas or injuries, physical effects, social and cultural environment. This knowledge is instilled in graduate schools of social work and are integrated into the skills of direct practice that are developed by the student for about two years of post-graduate experience under the supervision of a clinical social worker (CSW). This period is enough to prepare the clinical social worker to be able to practice independently with a license from the State as a professional clinical social worker. In the following years, clinical social workers can obtain more generalized practice or can decide to specialize in one or more areas of practice.

Clinical social work is important because of the skills of its practitioners to be able to adapt to different settings and functions, including head of team members in multidisciplinary centers and in community mental health centers. Clients/patients, individuals, couples, families, children and groups, benefit from a wide variety of direct services including but not limited to, psychosocial evaluations, treatment plans, crisis intervention, and case management. The skillful and flexible application of knowledge, theories, and methods of intervention with the psychosocial focus, is a seal of quality of clinical social work.

The direct process of interventions from person/people are conducted with people of all ages and of natural differences, from prevention services, crisis interventions, psychoeducational, up to the defense of the rights of clients/patients, as well as the extensive process of psychotherapy. Most often, clinical social workers supervise and consult with other colleagues and can also take part in direct and indirect practice (administration, research, and writing). It is a practice standard for clinical social workers to continue clinical education and adhere to the professional code of ethics (Center for Clinical Social Work Research, 2007).

Psychologists provide clinical counseling services, assess, and treat mental, emotional, and behavioral disorders. They use the science of psychology to treat complex human problems and promote change. They also promote resilience and help people discover their strengths. To become a licensed psychologist can take as little as eight years or as long as twelve years.

History of social work in the hospital setting:

Social work was introduced to hospitals in the United States by Dr. Richard Cabot in 1905. Dr. Cabot created the first position of social work in the world, giving it first to Garmet Pelton, and later was followed by Ida Cannon (Davidson, K., 1998). In 1918, The National Association of Social Workers (NASW) was set up with the purpose to improve the relation between formal education and practice in hospitals. The role of the social workers was to provide social services to those people in need. However, the administrators only wanted the social workers to evaluate the social needs of patients in order to relieve the doctors, and to avoid the abuse of the hospital by the patients (Davidson, K., 1990).

The social Worker in the hospital setting:

1. **Communicates:** emphasize communication between the medical personnel, patients, and their families, and makes sure that that their medical needs are met.
2. **Offers emotional support:** focusing on psychosocial issues and the emotional needs of patients and their families.

3. **Advocates:** for the patient's rights making sure that the hospital provides quality medical services.
4. **Links:** making sure that the available resources for the patients are adequate.
5. **Advices**: personalizing interactions and understands feelings attitudes and behaviors of patients and their families.
6. **Intervenes:** between patients, families, and medical personnel.
7. **Coordinates:** organizing services for patients upon their discharge from the hospital.
8. **Educates:** transmitting knowledge, and teaching about the patients' rights including medical decisions, and end of life issues

Based on the author's years of experience in the Bronx Lebanon Hospital (1989-2013), social workers do little or nothing to promote themselves and their clinical services. The skills, abilities and contributions are not clear to other health care professionals (doctors, nurses). For instance, the doctor or nurse may not know that it takes skills for the social worker to be in a room with a suffering patient even though he/she has received years of academic training. All the years of education training, however, go to the wayside when the clinical social worker is questioned and cannot explain his/her unique skill set is. This is odd, for doctors and nurses know what their skills set are.in this instance. As pointed out by Davidson (1990), and Cowles, L. A., 2000), hospital social work has developed a font of knowledge and has influenced patient care by promoting recognition of the psychosocial part of health care. Social workers in health care settings bring a person and family-centered model of care to assessment and treatment, which differs from the patient-focused medical model (Garcés, C., 2019).

This author's experience as a social worker in the hospital setting began in 1989 at Bronx Lebanon Hospital Center in the South Bronx, New York (presently Bronx Care), which is one of the poorest neighborhoods in the United States and is composed of people from all over the world. Also, the people of the South Bronx suffer from multiple medical problems such , asthma, diabetes, Aids, cholesterol, hypertension, obesity. There are also psychosocial and mental health problems such as, delinquency, drug and alcohol abuse, prostitution, homelessness, child and elderly abuse, domestic violence. According to the report from the Office of Census of the United States (2006), more than 38% of the population of the South Bronx live below the poverty level. The numbers are worse for children: 49% live in poverty (Bronx Lebanon Hospital Center, 2007).

Social workers work in hospitals, educating the medical staff about discharge planning, crisis interventions, hospice and palliative care, uniting patients, and families with available community resources. Clinical social workers collaborate with physicians and nurses and other medical staff (Miozrahi, T., Abramson, J., 1985., Garcés, C., 2002) to show the social needs of patients, not just the presenting problem. While the time of home visits is part of the past, clinical social workers continue taking part in evaluations of family situations, reinforcing social supports that are available for those patients who are discharged from the hospital and ere in need of continuing of care Garcés, C., 2002-2019). The clinical social worker contributes to the overall operation of the hospital setting by helping/assisting patients and their families cope with crisis, including death, and with the discharge planning process from the hospital.

The hospital social worker also:

1. Assess the social-environmental problems of patients
2. Help patients examine workable solutions to their social-environmental problems
3. Help/assists patients of community resources for their social-environmental problems
4. Contact community agencies to request services for their social-environmental problems of patients
5. Inform patients of how their medical problems may create social-environmental problems for them
6. Refers patients to proper hospital personnel for aid with their social-environmental problems

During the pandemic of Covid-19, clinical social workers have been performing their clinical roles with the discharge process outside the hospital, in their homes. Doctors and nurses need continued direct contact with patients. Because of the pandemic, hospitals had to reduce the amount of personnel who were considered "essential," among them were social workers. These regulations were imposed by the federal and local governments. The clinical social workers were not able to directly communicate with patients with Covid-19 and their families because of this mandate. Discharge planning is provided via telehealth session with patients and families.

A clinical social worker is a professional who holds a Master or Doctor degree in social work from an accredited school of social work. In addition to at least two years of post-master's supervised experience in a clinical setting. The social worker must be licensed, certified, or registered at the clinical level in the authority of practice. A clinical social worker provides direct services, including intrapsychic dynamics, and life management issues. Clinical social work services are based on biopsychosocial perspectives. Services consist of diagnosis, treatment (including psychotherapy and counseling), client centered advocacy, consultation, evaluation, and prevention of mental illness, emotional or behavioral disturbances.

Social workers can work as:

1. Administrators in community mental health clinics.
2. Researchers.
3. Rehabilitators.
4. In medical and psychiatric hospitals.
5. Case managers.
6. Psychotherapists.

Clinical social work is a specialty that meets the following requirements:

1. Has a systematic body of theories that sustains its work.
2. Has professional authority that emanates from the domain of theory.

3. Has community recognition that the profession is valid.
4. Has a code of ethics that governs the behavior of its members.
5. Has a consistent professional culture and professional vocabulary and method.

Clinical social work bases its method based on the knowledge derived from research and practice evaluation, including its own knowledge with a specific content. Also, recognizes the complexity of interactions between people and their environment, and the ability of people to react to multiple influences or circumstances upon themselves, including psychosocial health or environmental factors such as the Covid-19. Social work extracts from theories of human development, social and systems theories to analyze complex situations to get acquainted with individual changes within social and cultural organizations (NASW-Definition of Social Work, 2000).

The clinical social worker as family psychotherapist:

1. Teaches to all family members about how family's function in general, and how they work themselves.
2. Helps the family to focus less on the member that was identified as "problematic" and to focus more on the family.
3. Helps to name conflicts and anxieties. Also helps the family to develop strategies to solve them.
4. Strengthens all members to be able to work together in solving their problems.
5. Teaches ways to solve conflicts and changes within the family. Sometimes, the way members solve their problems and leads them to have more probability in developing depressive symptoms.

The knowledge base of clinical social work includes the theories of biology, psychological and sociological development, diversity and cultural competency, interpersonal relationships, family and group dynamics, emotional problems, addictions, impact of emotional problems on people, traumas. These knowledges are encouraged in the Graduate Schools of Social Work and are integrated in the skills of direct practice which are developed by the students for about two years of experience postgraduate under the supervision of a clinical social worker. This period of training is sufficient to prepare the clinical social worker to be able to practice in an autonomous way with license from the State as a clinical social worker. In the following years after graduation, clinical social workers can obtain a generalized advanced practice or can also decide to specialize in one or more areas.

Clinical social work is important because of the skills of its practitioners in adapting to distinct roles, including department heads in multidisciplinary centers, in hospitals (medical/psychiatric), and in community mental health centers. Clients/patients, individuals, couples, families, children the elderly, and groups receive help from a wide variety of direct services that are provided by clinical social workers, including psychosocial evaluations, treatment, crisis intervention, and case management. The skillful application of knowledge, theories, and methods of intervention, with the biopsychosocial approach, is a quality seal of clinical social work. The interventions of direct process from person/people, are conducted with people of all ages and different by nature, from preventive services, crisis intervention and psychoeducational services to the defense of patients' rights, as well as the short or extensive process of counseling and psychotherapy. Typically, clinical social workers supervise and consult with other colleagues and can also take part in direct and indirect practice (administration, research, writing). This is a practice norm for clinical social workers to take part and to continue a long and extensive career to continue their clinical education and adhere to the professional code of ethics (Center for Clinical Social Work Research, 2014).

The social work profession has evolved from philanthropy and the welfare theory to social technology, in recent terms, is considered as a scientific discipline in the development of social sciences, which guides a profession with a define space in the satisfaction of human needs, existentially (material), and appreciatively (affective and political). Clinical social work is reinventing and having meaning with respect to a holistic vision of its reality (NASW, 2014). With the arrival of globalization of financial markets, scientific and technological advance, clinical social workers ought to be thinking from a more comprehensive and interdisciplinary dimension, with new methods of intervention, where we can improve the welfare and wellbeing of people, families, and society.

Nonclinical social work:

The non-clinical social worker can incorporate psychotherapy in public or private organizations, and in case management. Many times, non-clinical social workers can work providing counseling and helping clients in finding employment, coordinating rehabilitation programs, prevention of child abuse/elderly abuse and neglect programs. Typically, this practice makes them collaborate with clients based in consultation (NASW, 2014).

How are psychiatric problems diagnosed?

According to the Desk reference to the Diagnostic Criteria (DSM-5 (2013):

1. A medical history of the client/patient is necessary.
2. Physical exam and lab work.
3. Psychiatric, psychological, or psychosocial evaluation, which has questions about thoughts, feelings, and behavior.

Wrong ideas about what is meant by clinical social worker/psychotherapist:

To better understand what a psychotherapist means, first we must talk about what it is not. There are many ideas and wrong concepts about the meaning of psychotherapist. Some of them include:

1. **Wrong Ideas: The clinical social worker/psychotherapist is like a friend to whom people pay to listen:**
   To think that the clinical social worker/psychotherapist is a friend who is hired, discount the amount of education and professional training that is needed to better the mental health

of people that we serve. Most clinical social workers/psychotherapists have six years of education. Others have more than a decade of professional studies.

2. **Wrong Ideas: The clinical social worker/psychotherapist tells people what to do:** Most clinical social workers/psychotherapists do not tell anybody what they must do. They are not like their parents, teachers, or trainers. They do not dictate or yell instructions to follow. Clinical social workers/psychotherapists collaborate with people to whom they teach skills to be able to live a healthy life and be able to make good decisions. Clinical social workers/psychotherapists empower people and try not to create dependency.

3. **Wrong Ideas: The clinical social worker/psychotherapist, reads the mind:** The clinical social worker/psychotherapist does not try to guess what the client/patient is thinking or analyzes his/her ideas. The main concern of the clinical social worker/psychotherapist is in what the client/patient is thinking, only because he/she wants to help.

Five theories that describe clinical social work practice (Engard, B., 2017).

1. **Psychosocial Theory.** Its focus is on the way that people are molded and how they react to their environment.
2. **Psychodynamic Theory.** Tries to understand the behavior of people.
3. **Transpersonal Theory.** Was influenced by Carl Jung, uses positive influences, instead of human illnesses, and defenses for the realization human potential. This theory uses saints, artists, heroes, and other similar figures people who have a good ego can try to emulate as role models and aspirations.
4. **Learning Cognitive Theory.** Its focus is on the effects of the environment, and reinforces behavior, however, Bandura, A (1977) added two important dimensions: Mediating forces follow between the stimulus and the answer, and people can learn behavior trough observation.
5. **Systems Theory.** Claims that behavior is influenced by a variety of factors that work together as a system. Parents, friends, school, social status, home environment, and other factors influence how a person thinks and behaves.

Guides for the intervention of people with mental health problems:

1. Be respectful.
2. Be calm, clear, and direct in the communication.
3. Be consistent and predictable.
4. Establish limits, rules, and expectations
5. Maintain professional distance
6. Accept the client/patient as he/she is
7. Attributing symptoms to the disease
8. Do not take symptoms of the illness as personal
9. Maintain a cheerful outlook even during failure

10. Acknowledge and praise positive behavior
11. Help the client to make realistic goals and objectives
12. Have the attitude of "I don't know" to tough questions

Ethical and professional values:

According to the National Association of Social Workers (NASW, 2002), code of ethics are standards of moral behavior for a society or group, such as social workers. The code of ethics for a profession has standards of behavior for a certain profession. These ethical codes reflect concerns and define basic principles that helps as a professional guidance. Its purpose is:

1. provides a practical position to help professionals in making decisions towards clients/ patients and society,
   a. guarantees society that the professionals are going to show sensibility with respect to social expectations,
   b. guarantees the professionals respect of their integrity and freedom,
   c. aids in clarifying responsibilities that the professionals have towards the clients/ patients,
2. Social workers need to evaluate the ethical practice in the following considerations:
   a. The professional moral judgement (do not make the client/patient uncomfortable).
   b. Legal aspects (laws that govern).
   c. Ethical implications (apply ethical principles that should be respected).
3. This code of ethics is divided in five sections:
   a. the main goal is to help people in need and to focus on their problems,
   b. social justice; challenging social injustice,
   c. dignity and courage of the person. Respect for the individual.
   d. Importance of human relationships,
   e. integrity: practice within the area of expertise and commitment to better professional skills.

To remember and consider:

1. The needs of clients/patients.
2. Level of professional competency of the clinical social worker.
3. Clinical orientation of the clinical social worker.
4. Cultural competence of the clinical social worker with the client/patient.
5. Clinical social workers should respect the code of professional ethics.

Elements to succeed as a clinical social worker:

1. **Removing the language barrier:** Communication is essential to diagnosing mental health problems, so understanding what clients/patients express is critical. The use of interpreters

may help, but a clinical social worker who speaks the client's/patient's native language, and can understand cultural nuances and jargon, is often effective.

2. **Collaboration with primary care physicians:** Collaborating with primary care physicians is vital to reaching the Latino population.

3. **Encouraging family involvement:** Latinos have strong family support system. Family support can ease the stigma of mental health problems and encourages client/s/patients to address it. Sharing information with family members increases their understanding of the problem and helps them better to support the client/patient.

4. **Providing sensitive, culturally competent treatment:** An adequate intervention with clients/patients who only speak Spanish needs an understanding of both languages, also requires the skills to communicate efficiently in either language at various levels. Problems in evaluating client's/patient's mental health problems could happen when there is a lack of understanding of ethnic, cultural, social, and economic contents which are important for the understanding of attitudes about the social needs and behavior. Difficulty in making assessments can also occur when the clinical social worker does not have the proper training for interventions in mental health.

5. **Educating about the physiologic roots of mental illness:** Lack of information and misunderstandings would worsen the stigma. Informing details about the psychiatric diagnosis, discussing treatment plans, and answering questions could be the best way to end stigma. Explaining the biological and environmental causes of mental illness is educational to many Latinos.

6. **Empathy:** Is the ability to identify with an understanding the point of view of other people's experiences. The National Association of Social Workers (NASW, 2003), defines empathy "as the act of perceiving, understanding, experiences, and responding to another person's emotional state of ideas." Putting oneself in someone's shoes and recognizing those world experiences, perceptions, points of view, and unique views that allows clinical social workers to understand and build together strong relationships with clients/patients. This is a vital skill that helps clinical social workers decide the needs of clients/patients, based on their unique experiences to be able to provide efficient professional services (Barker, R.L., 2003).

7. **Communication:** (verbal/nonverbal), Is a vital skill for clinical social workers. The ability to communicate clearly with a wide variety of people is essential. In addition to being aware to body language and other nonverbal signs. This means having to communicate proper and efficiently with clients/patients regardless of their cultural history, age, sexual orientation, intellectual level, physical or emotionally disability. Clinical social workers should also communicate effectively with other health care providers, colleagues, and agencies, and should clearly document and report adequate information.

8. **Organization:** Clinical social workers have a busy schedule of responsibilities to others, to serve and support multiple clients/patients, including documentation, bill reports, and collaboration. This requires that clinical social workers must be organized and be able to prioritize the needs of clients/patients to manage their caseloads.

Disorganization and poor administration of time can cause the clinical social worker not to provide adequate attention to the needs of the clients/patients and can result in negative consequences.

9. **Critical thinking:** Is the ability to be able to analyze information obtained without inclined preferences of observation and communication. Clinical social workers should have the ability to evaluate each case by collecting information through interviews and research. Thinking critically and without prejudice, and making adequate decisions, finding resources, and formulating proper intervention plans for clients/patients.

10. **Listening carefully:** Is necessary for clinical social workers to be able to understand and identify needs of clients/patients. Listening carefully, concentrating, asking proper questions, using techniques such as paraphrasing and summarizing, also helps to build a trusting relationship with clients/patients.

11. **Personal attention:** Clinical social work can be demanding and emotionally stressful. It is important for the clinical social workers to take part in activities that will help them to reduce stress and improve their personal wellbeing. Doing these activities helps to prevent emotional exhaustion, fatigue and is crucial for a sustainable career. By paying attention to their own self, clinical social workers will be able to offer the best services to their clients/patients.

12. **Cultural competence:** Working effectively with clients/patients from diverse cultural backgrounds requires to be respectful and respond to diverse cultural and political beliefs. Clinical social workers should have knowledge and respect for cultural histories, and as stablish by the National Association of Social Workers (NASW, 2003), examine their own cultural history, while seeking necessary knowledge, skills and values that can improve the provision of services to people with a variety of cultural experiences associated with race, ethnicity, education, social class, sexual orientation, religion, age, or disability. By having critical attitude and appreciation for diversity and value for individual differences, it helps clinical social workers to provide professional services to people with what they need.

13. **Professional commitment:** Being a successful clinical social worker requires a long life of learning. Clinical social workers must have a professional commitment to values and ethics and continue to develop professional competence. This commitment is necessary to achieve the mission of social work, "to improve human wellbeing and help meet the basic human needs of all people, with particular attention to the needs of empowering vulnerable, oppressed and living in poverty.

14. **Advocacy:** Clinical social workers promote social justice and empower clients/patients and communities through support. The ability to support and skill allows clinical social workers to stand for and argue for their clients/patients and connect them with resources and opportunities that are necessary, especially when clients/patients are vulnerable or cannot advocate for themselves (NASW, 2003).

Conclusion and recommendations:

Social work is a profession that is advancing in a way that governments and employers around the world are acknowledging the tremendous impact that clinical social workers have with people they serve in their communities. Less crime, better results in medical and mental health system, more people having access to employment and education are the result of social work, supporting people to have control of their own future and make reality their aspirations. As a profession based on human rights, social work has an essential role in society advocating for communities to raise their voices and defend their rights along with others. The strength of the profession lies in its ability to build participatory democracy, uniting communities in sustainable futures and to defend human rights.

Clinical social workers have a key role, thus raising the voices of people whose worries are not always heard proportioned. People outside the social work profession have the possibility of not being familiarized or informed about the psychotherapeutic services clinical social workers provide. Lack of knowledge and understanding of what clinical social workers do in the hospital setting and in community mental health centers do may create conflicts in the collaboration with other professionals in providing clinical services. The efficient intervention of clinical social workers depends, in part, on how other health care professionals and the public perceive the role of the clinical social worker. The modern clinical social worker must adapt to the globalized world, where the institutions are affecting the unilateral rules and its practice. The progressive increase of different social cultural consumers, especially in hospitals and community mental health centers, constitute a challenge for clinical social workers.

Clinical social workers help people to receive quality care and the needed resources to live a quality life. Aiding children with special needs in schools, aiding people with terminal illness, with changes in their everyday lives, and providing needed psychotherapy services to people with emotional problems. As clinical social workers we serve in society in diverse ways. While it is a requirement the use of techniques to help people with diverse medical, psychological, and psychosocial problems, as clinical social workers we could benefit by making use of the comprehensive approach.

Anxiety and depression around the world have increased due to the pandemic of Covid- 19 (Coronavirus), which has brought in fear and uncertainty among the population. For people with mental health problems, there is an increased risk of these conditions. Now that some places have been opening to the public (shopping malls, restaurants, stores, etc..), people are returning to their "normal way of life." However, those people with emotional problems could face serious problems adjusting. How can them go through the challenges of continuing their daily lives? How can their family and friends help them? How can clinical social workers help them?

Stigma surrounding mental health exists globally. However, according to limited available research, this stigma may be especially strong in Latin American countries and communities. It is this author's advice that people affected by mental health stigma, either directly or indirectly, may consider addressing this with their loved ones and seeking help from culturally competent mental health professionals. Aiding Latinos overcome their stigma about mental illness is not easy. The more that clinical social workers understand about Latino culture the better.

The challenge for clinical social workers is to be able to prove their professional and clinical skills, to be able to better the emotional and social well-being of the people they serve. Clinical social workers should contribute to initiatives of research, not only to be able to prove Their efficiency in the psychotherapeutic interventions, but also to promote knowledge and understanding among other colleagues about the importance of finding and communicating the psychosocial and mental health needs of the people who receive professional services. Also, clinical social workers ought to understand that they play a key role by showing the traumatic stress and emotional relationships when a person is diagnosed with mental illness and the stigma that comes along with it. As clinicians, social workers play a key role because they are the ones who shape the cultural sensitivity of any prevention program in their professional life. Thus, the beliefs of social workers' values, world vision, and ways of knowing are essential components efforts to provide services that are authentic and culturally sensitive.

Cultural competence should be a requirement for clinical social workers and other mental health professionals who work with culturally diverse clients/patients. Cultural competency will improve the quality of mental health for people of different ethnic groups.

Population	Language, Education and Poverty
2000 US Census: Latinos were 52.1% of the population of East Harlem, New York, in "El Barrio" as it is referred by the Latino residents.	**US Census Bureau (2016), in the State of New York:** 83% of Latinos do not Speak English in their homes.
2005 Statistical data of Latinos in the United States: 14% of the total population of New York State	23.5% of Latinos has completed less of nine years of high school compared to 6.3% of the general population, 3% of White and 5.4% of African Americans
Pew Hispanic Center report (2015): 25% Latinos of the total population of New York State	**Academic education:** only 12% of Latinos have graduated from a university, compared to the general population, 31.1% of Whites and 17%.7% of African Americans.
New York Controller's Office (2016): almost one in every New Yorker identifies themselves as Latino or Hispanic. Between 1990 and 2014- Latino population in New York State has increased 66%, reaching almost 3.7 million (19%) of the population, and most of them live in New York City Metropolitan area.	**Adult Latinos in New York City, between the ages of 25 and more:** 35% did not graduated from high school, compared to the 14% among adult Latinos
The US Bureau of Census (2018): expects the adult Latino population to grow about 55% in the next three decades, compared with the rest of the White population. -estimates that for next 2030 there will be 74.81 million of Latinos in the United States.	**Poverty rate:** was 23.4% compared to White people or 12.4%, Afro-Americans 226.2%, Native Americans 27.6%, meanwhile Asians were 12.3%.

References

Abramson, J. S., Mizrahi, T. (1996). When Social Workers and Physicians Collaborate: Positive and negative interdisciplinary experiences. Journal of the National Association of Social Workers, 4, 2-28.

Anderson, S., & Sabatelli, R. (1999). Family interaction: A multigenerational development perspective. (2nd ed.). Needham Heights, MA: Allyn & Bacon.

American Psychological Association (1979-1988). What is Psychotherapy? In Bloch Sidney (Ed). An Introduction to the Psychotherapist. Oxford University Press, p. 92-92.

Bureau of US Census. American Fact Finder-Results. Factfinder.census.gov. Retrieved January 16-2020.

Bandura, A. (1997). Social Learning Theory. New York General Learning Press.

Betancourt, J. R. (2001). Cultural Competence. Marginal or Mainstream Movement? New England Journal of Medicine; 351: 953-955.

Campinha-Bacote, J. (1998). A Model and Instrument for Addressing Cultural Competence in Health Care. Journal of Nursing Education; 38 (5), 204-207. Google Scholar.

Carter, R. (Ed), (1999). Addressing Cultural Issues in Organizations. Beyond the Corporate Context. Thousand Oaks, CA: Sage Publications.

Guarnaccia, P. J. (2008). Panic attacks in the Latino population: Culturally bound and distinct from panic attacks?

Center for Clinical Social Work (2007). What is the Difference Between Clinical and Non-Clinical Social Work? American Board of Examiners in Clinical Social Work.

Comas-Diaz, L. (1995). Puerto Ricans and sexual child abuse. In L.A. Fontes (Ed.), Sexual abuse in nine North American cultures: treatment and prevention (pp.31-66). Thousands Oaks, CA: Sage Publications.

Davis, L., & Proctor, E. (1989). Race as an issue in practice. In race, gender & class: Guidelines for practice with individuals, families, and groups (pp. 1-9). Englewood Cliffs, Prentice- Hall, INC.

Coon, D. (2001). Introduction to Psychology. Gateways to Mind and Behavior. Nineth edition. Warthworth.

Davidson, K. (1990). Role Blurring and the Social Worker's Search for a Clear Domain. Health and Social Work, 15, 228-234.

Desk Reference to the Diagnostic Criteria From DSM-5. American Psychiatric Association Publishing. Washington DC, London-England.

Dillon, F. R., De La Rosa, G. E., Ibáñez, J. (2013). Acculturative Stress and Diminishing Family Cohesion Among Latino Immigrants. Springer.

Diaz Christina, J. J., Niño, Michael (2019). Familism and the Hispanic Health Advantage: The role of Immigrants status. Sage Journals.

Engard, Brian. (2017). 5 Social Work Theories that inform practice. Social Work Helper.

Fernández, R. L., Das, Amar, K., Weissman, César Alfonso Myrna (2005-2011). Depression in US Hispanics: Diagnostic and Management Considerations in Family Practice. The Journal of The American Board of Family Practice, 18 (4), 282-296.

Garcés, C. M. (2002). The Social Worker in the Emergency Room. Doctoral Dissertation. Yeshiva University (WWSSW). New York.

Garcés, C. M. (2018). La Intervención del Trabajador Social en el Centro Hospitalario-Retos para la Profesión. Edición Revisada Palibrio Publishing Company.

Garcés, C. M. (2019). Hospital Social Work Interventions. Gold Touch Publisher.

Giachello, A. (1999). Hispanic Health Rx. University of Chicago. Chicago Journal. Volume 98, Issue 5.

Gelman, C. (2004). Empirically based principles for culturally competent practice with Latinos. Journal of Ethics & Cultural Diversity. 13 (1), 83-108.

Green, J. (1999). Cultural Awareness in the Human Services. 3rd.ed. Englewood Cliffs, NJ. Prince Hall.

Gomez, A. Beloz, J. Altern, J. (2001). The Botanicals as a Culturally Appropriate Health Care Option for Latinos.,

Gutiérrez, L., Yeakley, A., & Ortega, R. (2000). Educating students for social work with Latinos: Issues for the new millennium. Journal of Social Work Education. 36, 5541-557.

Heyck, D. (1994). Barrios and borderlands: Cultures of Latinos and Latinas in the United States. New York: Routledge.

Hispanics in the US (2006). Census Bureau, Population Estimates.

Insel, T. R. ((2008). Assessing the Economic Cost of Serious Mental Illness. The American Journal of Psychiatry. 165 (6), 633-665.

Kim, D. (1999). Culturally Competence Practice. Pacific Grove, CA: Books/Cole.

Nathan Kline Institute Center of Excellence in Culturally Competent Mental Health (2019). Evidenced Based Practices in Support of Cultural Competence in Mental Health Services.

Lewis, M. J., West, B., Bautista, L., Greenberg, A., Done-Pérez, I. (2005). Perceptions of Service Providers and community members on intimate partner violence within a Latino community. Health Education & Behavior. 32:69-83 (PubMed).

Lum, D. (1999). Cultural Competence Practice. Pacific Grove, CA: Books/Cole.

Melville. L. M. (2012). On Culture.: Edward B. Tyler's Primitive Culture (1871). BRANCH: Britain, Representation and Ninteenth-Century History. Ed. Dino Franco Felluga. Extension of Romantisism and Victorianism on the Net. Web (2022).

Williams R. (1958). Culture and Society. Colunbia University Press.

Navarro Vásquez, C. (2014). Pew Research Center Analysis of Decennial Census and American Community Survey (IPUMS).

National Association of Social Workers (2002). NASW Code of Ethics of The National Association of Social Workers. Washington DC: author.

National Association of Social Workers (2007). Definition of Clinical Social Work. Washington DC: Author.

National Association of Social Workers (2012). NASW Clinical and Non-Clinical Social Work. Washington DC: Author.

National Association of Social Workers (2014). NASW History of Psychiatric Social Work. Washington DC: Author.

National Association of Social Workers (2016). NASW Standards for Social Work Practice in Health care Settings. Washington DC: Author.

National Institute of Mental Health (2009-2012). Mental health. NAMI Latino Multicultural Action Center.

Ortega, A. N., Rosenheck, R., Alegría, M. Desai, R. A. (2000). Acculturation and the Lifetime Risk of Psychiatric and Substance Use Disorder Among Hispanics. J Nerv Ment Dis. 188 (11); 728-35. PubMed.

Pew Research Center (2014). Analysis of Decennial Census and American Community Survey (IPUMS).

Porto Pérez, J., Merino, M. (2017-2019). Definición de Curandero. (https://definicion. de.curandero/).

Uribe, R.M. Mora, O. L, Cortèz, A. R. (2007). Voces del estigma. Percepción del estigma en pacientes y familias con enfermedad mental. Universitas Médica. 48 (3) Retrieved 8/12/2021.

John Hopkins-Medicine (2019). Psychiatry and Behavioral Sciences: The History of Psychiatric Social Work.

The Hispanic Community in New York State (2016). Thomas, P., DiNapoli, New York state Comptroller. Nearly One in Five New Yorkers Identify as Hispanic or Latino.

Uribe, R.M., Mora, O.L., Cortez, A.R., (2007). Voces del estigma. Percepción del estigma en pacientes y familias con enfermedad mental. Universitas Medica. 48)3). Retrieved 0812/2021

Vega, W. A., López, S. R. (2001). Priority Issues in Latino Mental Health Services Research. Mental Health Research, Vol. 3, No. 4.

Walker, S., Beckett, C. (2004-2005). Social Work Assessment and Intervention. Russel House Publishing Company.

World Health Organization (2014). Mental Health: A State of Wellbeing: Author.

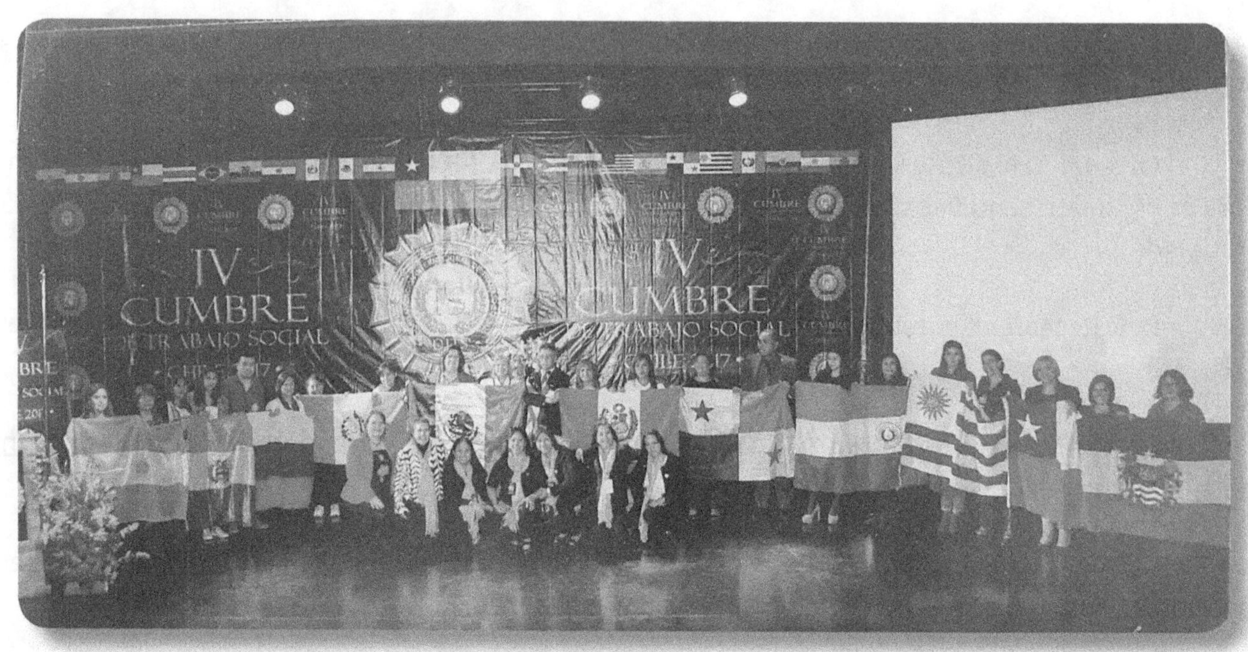

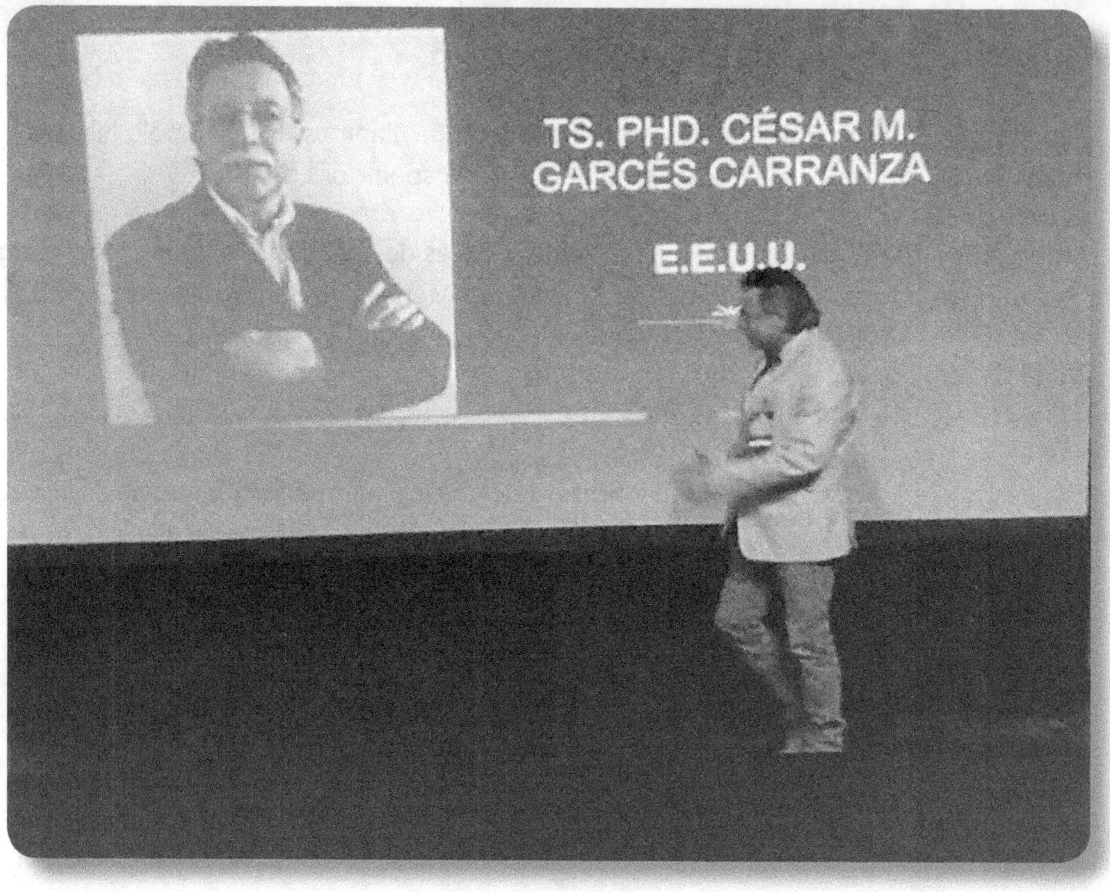
TS. PHD. CÉSAR M.
GARCÉS CARRANZA

E.E.U.U.

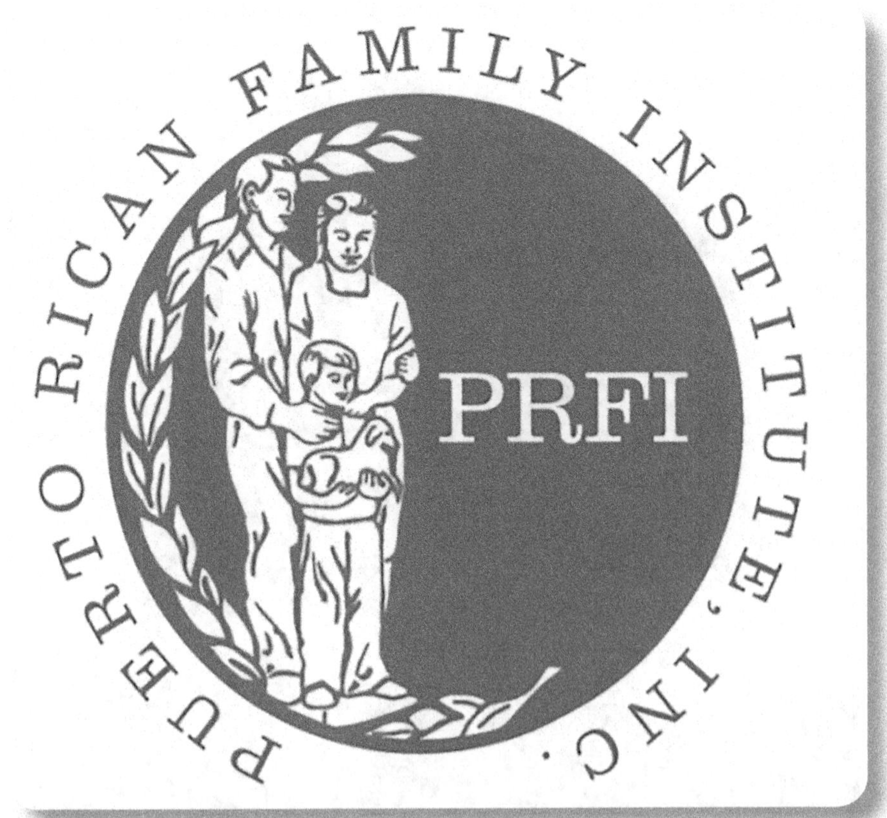

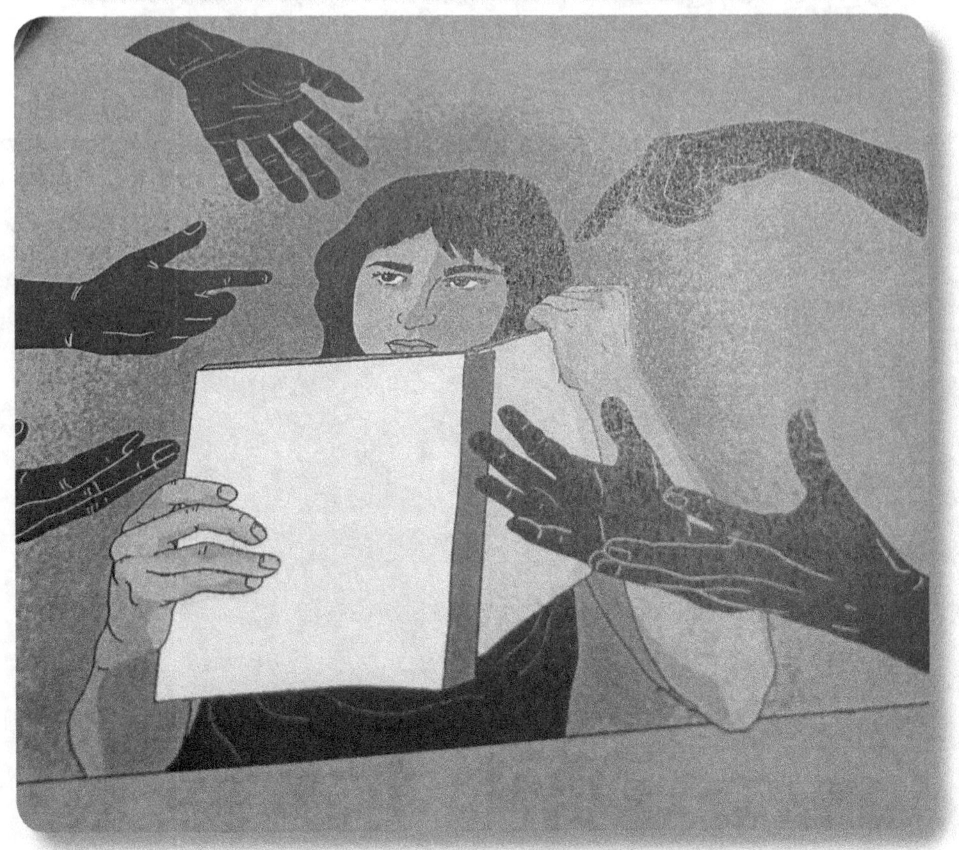

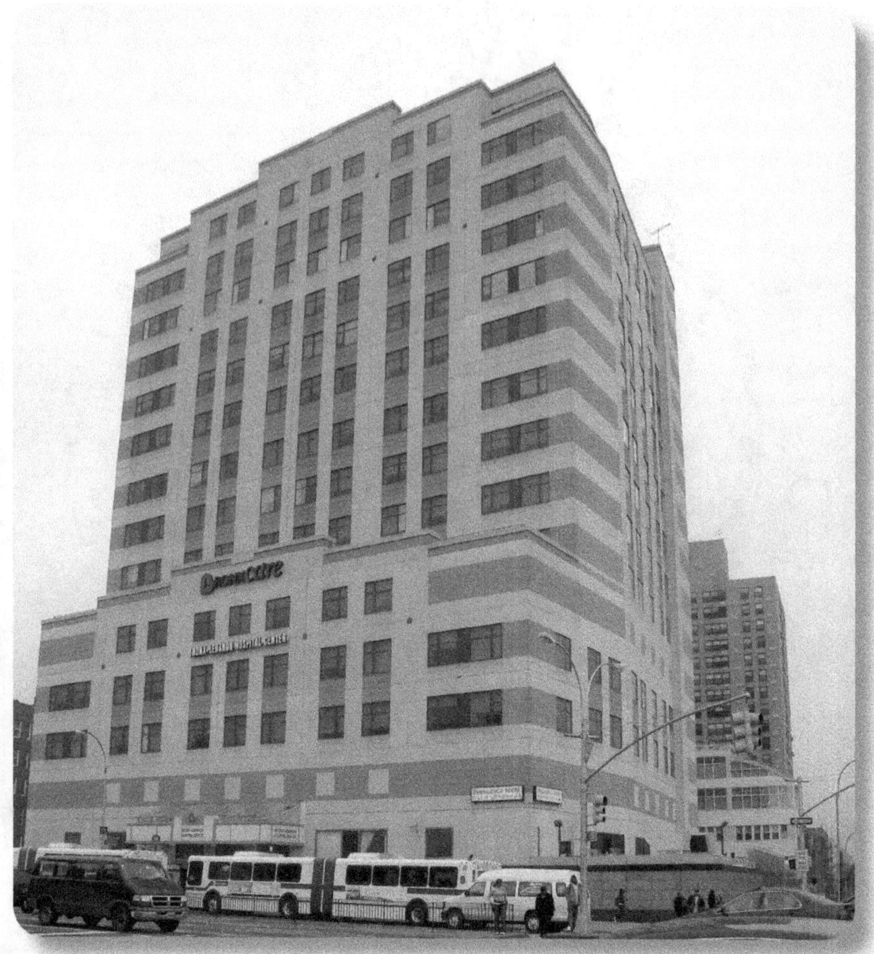

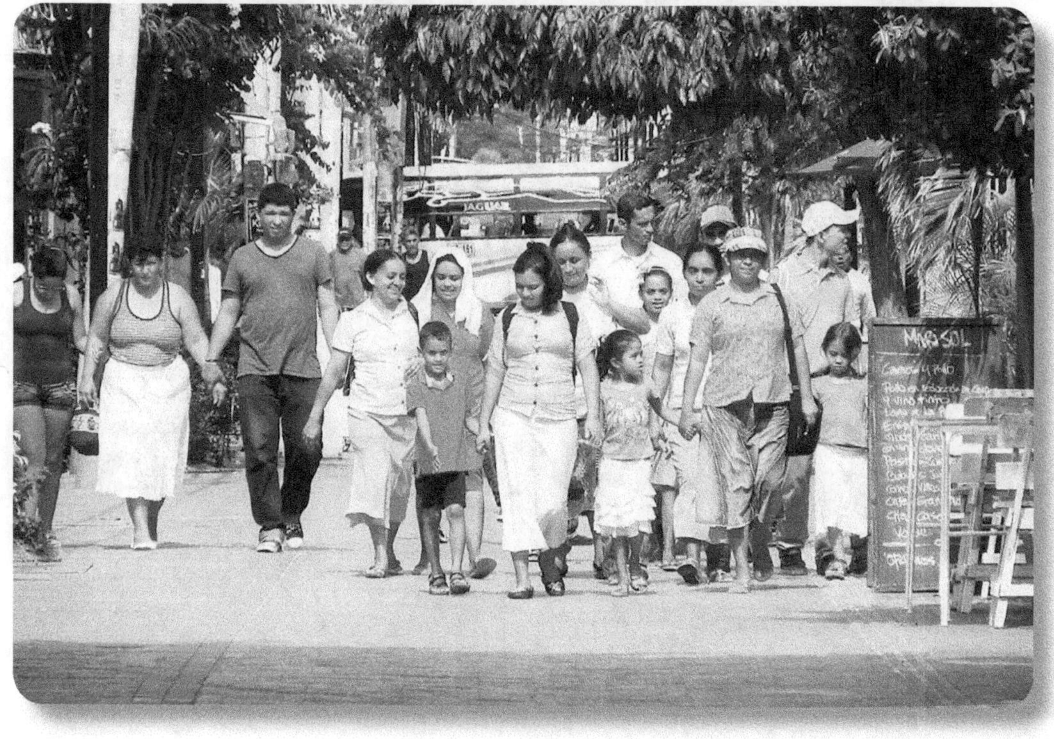

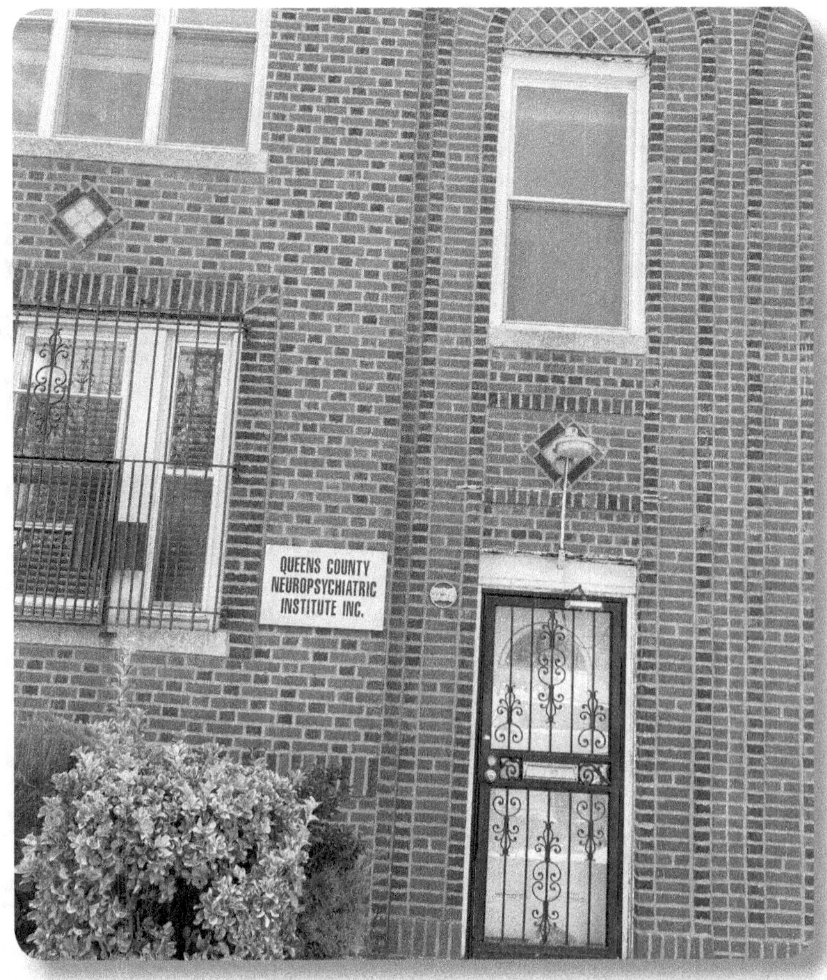
QUEENS COUNTY
NEUROPSYCHIATRIC
INSTITUTE INC.

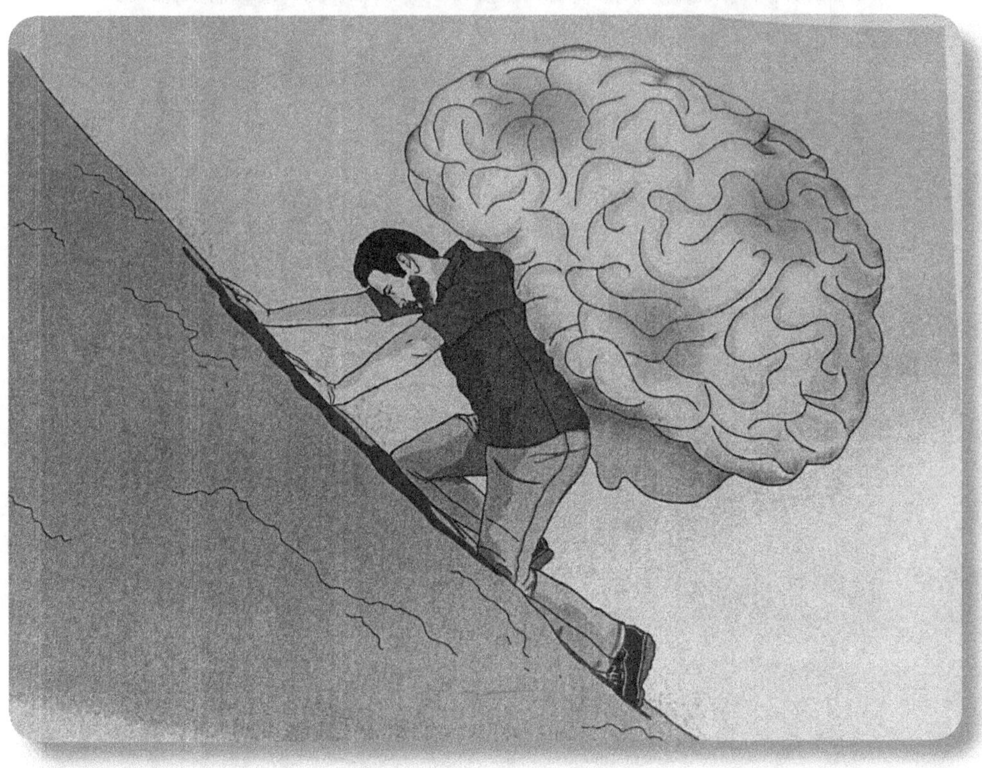

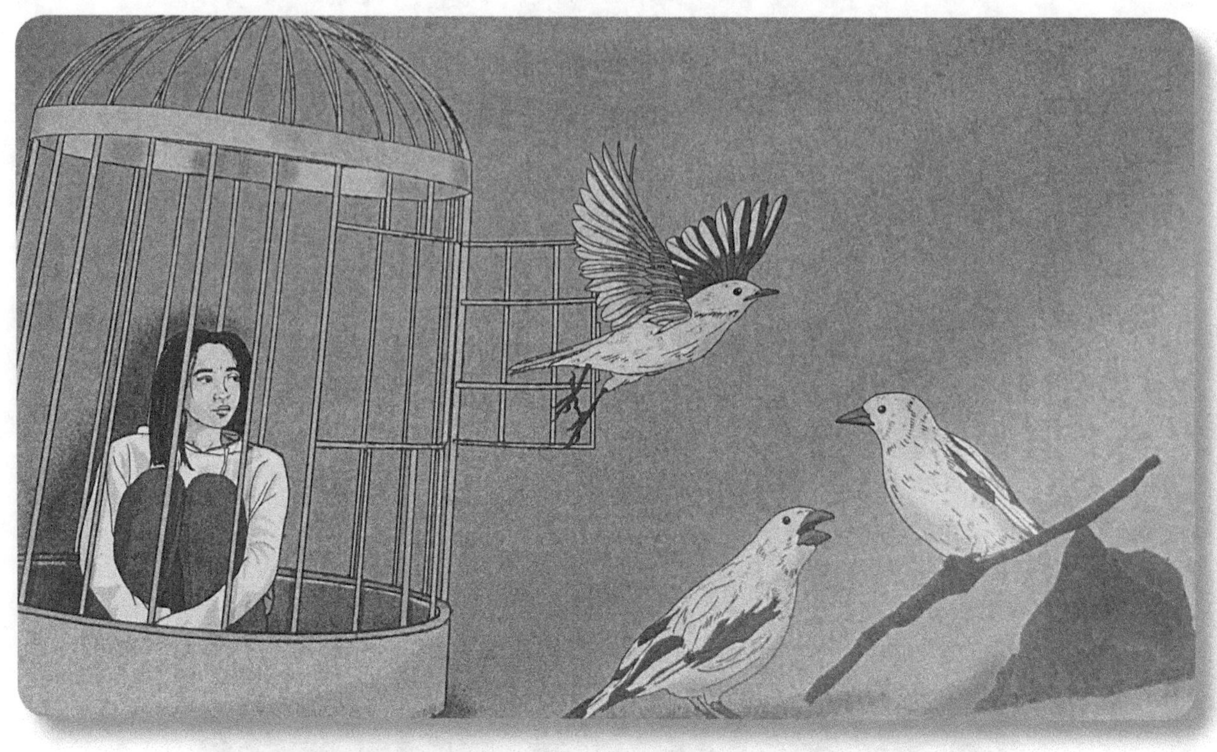

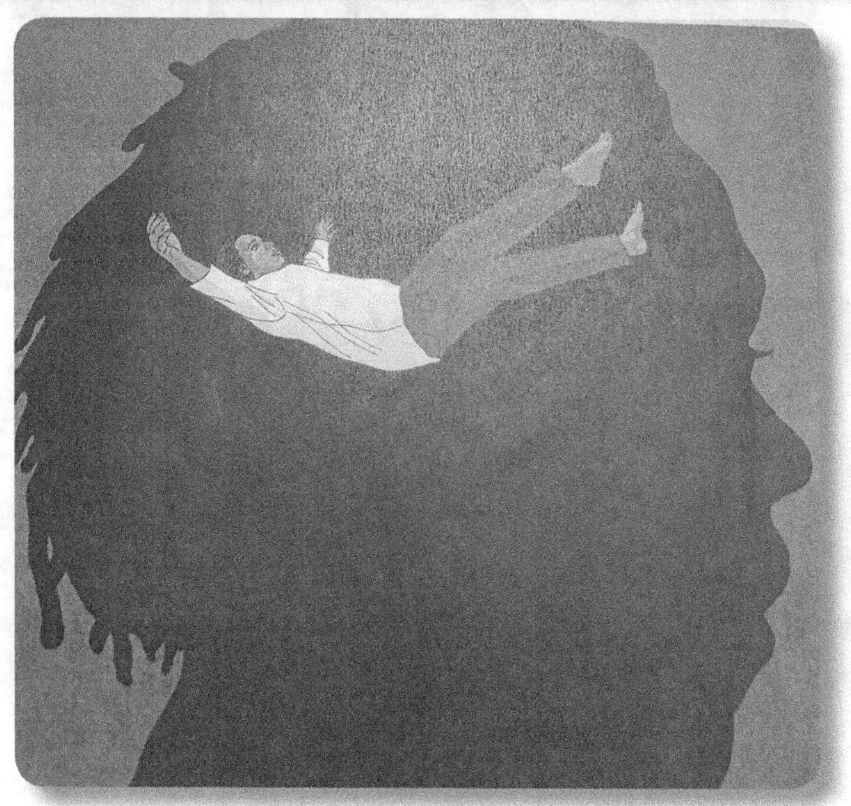

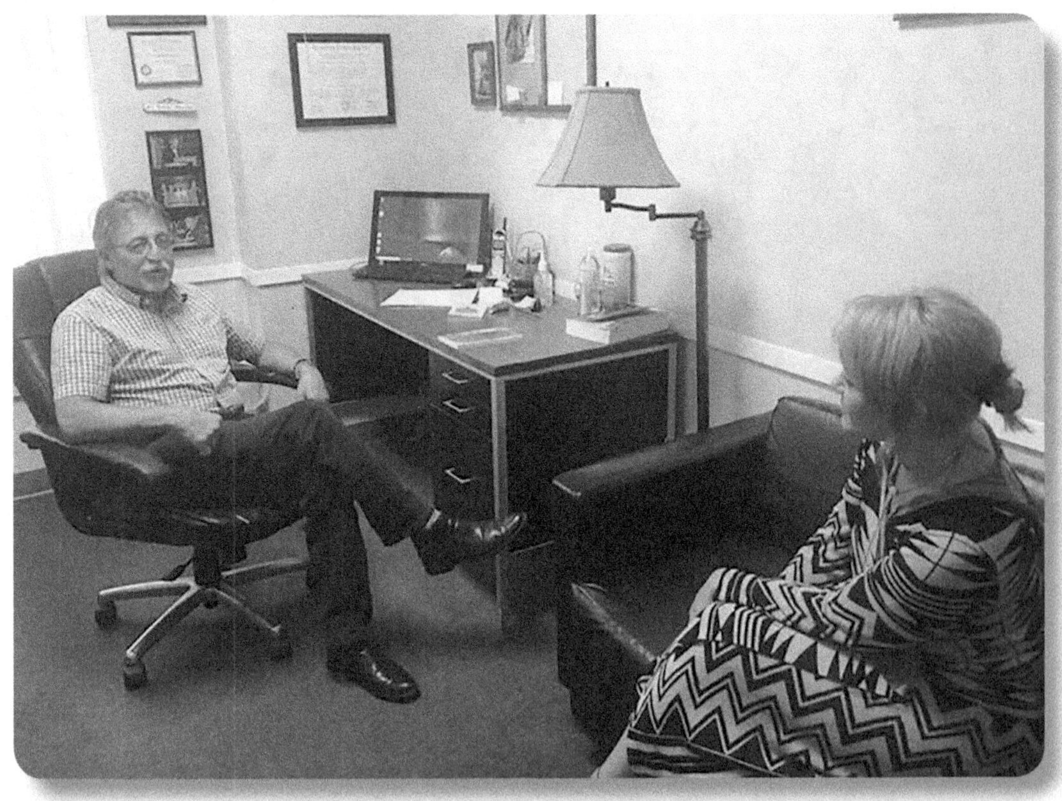

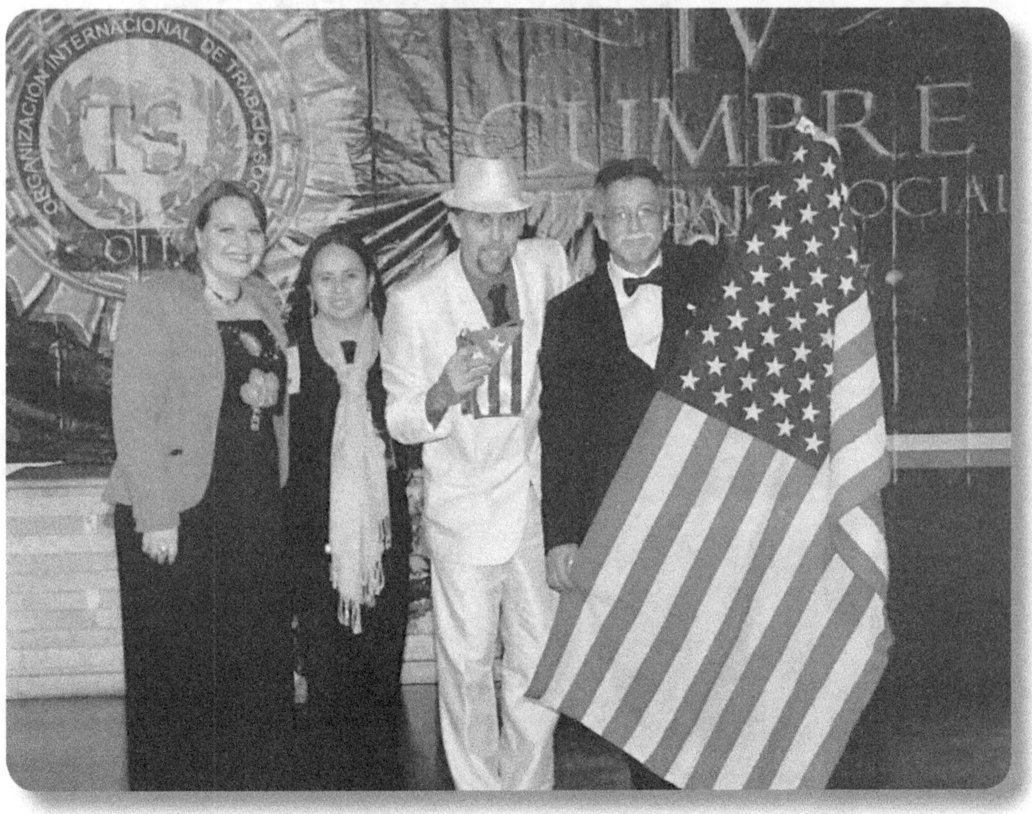

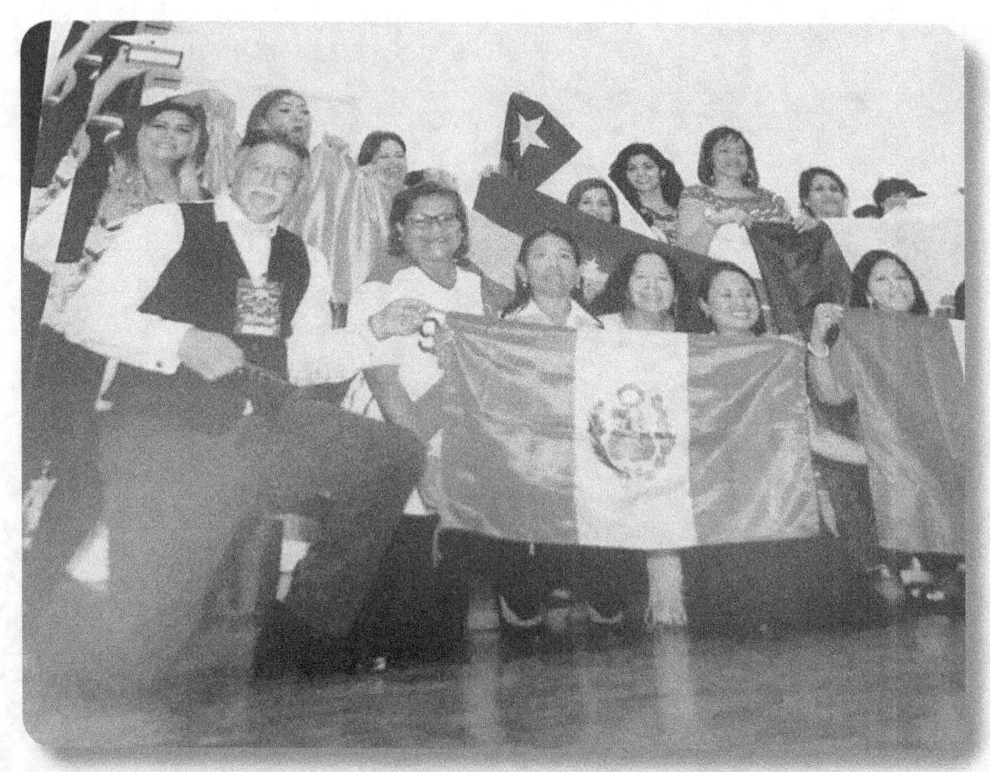

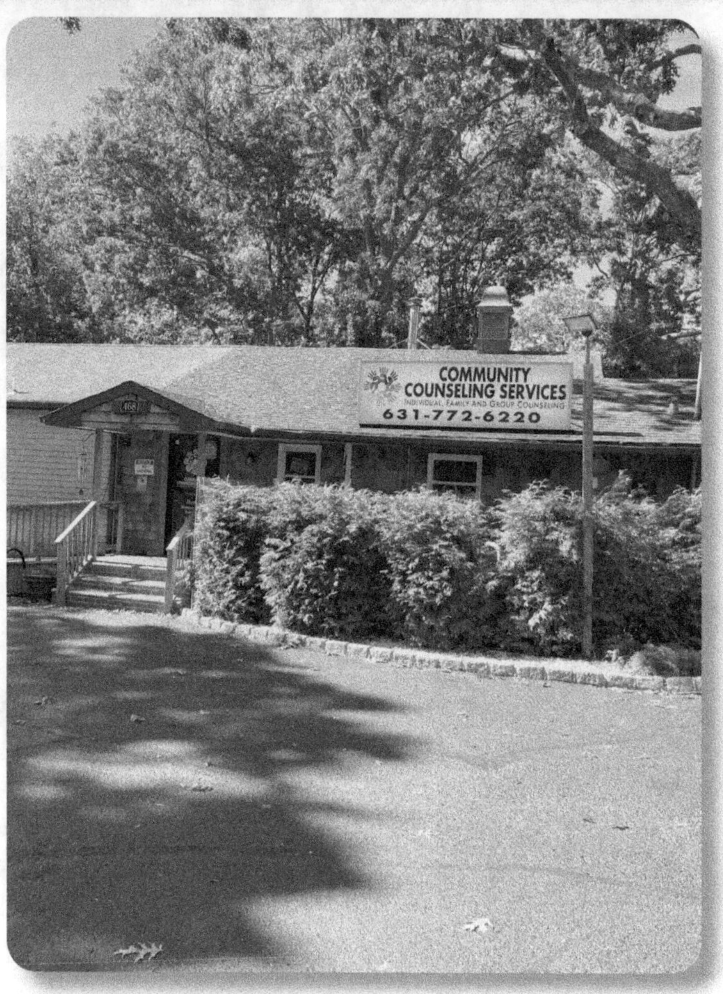

COMMUNITY
COUNSELING SERVICES
INDIVIDUAL, FAMILY AND GROUP COUNSELING
631-772-6220

Trabajo Social Cínico con Latinos en New York USA

César M. Garcés Carranza, PhD.

Dedicación

A mis hijos

Nicholas y Rachel

INDICE

Reconocimiento

Es siempre buena idea rendir tributo a las personas que nos ayudan en la creación y elaboración de nuestros proyectos. Es por esto que rindo tributo a:

Mi familia,

A mis colegas y amigos quienes indirecta y directamente contribuyeron en la

elaboración de mi libro "trabajo Social Clínico con Latinos en New york-USA.

A mis pacientes quienes siguen siendo inspiración en mi trayectoria profesional en salud mental. Curiosamente, ellos continúan ayudándome a crecer intelectual y personalmente. Sin los clientes/pacientes, no sabría las cosas que a diario aprendo.

":Muchas de las lecciones acerca de la vida vienen del reconocimiento de cómo otras personas de diferentes culturas ven las cosas."   *Edgard h. Schein.*

César M. Garcés Carranza, PhD.

Trabajo Social Clínico con Latinos

en Nueva York, USA \

César M. Garcés Carranza, PhD.

Agosto-2021

Resumen:

Hablar de salud mental en la comunidad Latina en New York es considerado como tabú. Esto implica decir que los padres, hijos y maestros de escuela no hablan de este tema lo suficiente. Algunas personas pueden considerar como inadecuado hablar de problemas de salud mental fuera de casa por temor al qué dirán.

Las experiencias del autor ejerciendo la práctica de trabajo social clínico con Latinos y personas de otros grupos minoritarios en New York es extensa. El autor trata de describir el contexto real del trabajo social clínico con Latinos, describiendo las principales áreas de la práctica profesional y la educación necesaria para ejercer esta especialidad. Los puntos principales de esta exploración personal descansan en una reflexión que pretende explicar las ventajas de ser un trabajador social clínico bilingüe y multicultural. Finalmente, hará algunas recomendaciones y sugerencias para el movimiento Latinoamericano de trabajo social clínico que ha estado creciendo durante los últimos años.

La historia del autor es la de una epopeya personal, de una búsqueda intensa. Como muchos inmigrantes, dejó su ciudad natal, Lima, Perú , para inmigrar a los Estados unidos. No fue fácil, seguramente, tener que lidiar con una nueva cultura, un nuevo idioma y con todas las peripecias que los inmigrantes experimentan en su afán de labrarse un futuro.

Como una forma de invitación, los trabajadores sociales clínicos deben contribuir a las iniciativas de investigación, no sólo para demostrar su eficacia en sus intervenciones terapéuticas, sino también para promover el reconocimiento y la aceptación de otros colegas de trabajo social clínico en el campo de la salud física y la salud mental. Los trabajadores sociales clínicos deben entender que juegan una función importante identificando y tratando una serie de problemas de salud mental, que abarcan desde el estrés postraumático hasta las reacciones emocionales que sufren las personas cuando se enfrentan a problemas relacionados con la salud mental. Como profesión que se basa en los derechos humanos, la especialidad del trabajo social clínico tiene una función esencial en todas las sociedades, facilitando que las comunidades alcen su voz y defiendan sus derechos junto con los demás. El poder del trabajo social clínico descansa en su propia base profesional, lo que implica su capacidad para crear una democracia participativa, para vincular a las comunidades en futuros sostenibles y proteger los derechos humanos.

Palabras-clave:

Latino, trabajo social, trabajo social clínico, trabajo social psiquiátrico, latino, salud mental, clínicas comunitarias de salud mental, hospital, estigma, cultura.

Durante los últimos 36 años, el Doctor Garcés ha estado ejerciendo como trabajador social clínico en el entorno hospitalario (sala de emergencias, unidades de cuidados intensivos, unidades médico-quirúrgicas, planificación de alta) y en clínicas psiquiátricas comunitarias en Nueva York, Jackson Heights, Queens y Long Island, New York con personas de diferentes grupos sociales, étnicos y multiculturales, especialmente con las comunidades Latinoamericanas. Como trabajador social clínico, este autor puede identificar los principales problemas psicosociales y emocionales, incluidas las intervenciones de crisis, proporcionar asesoramiento y explorar alternativas para identificar y aplicar alternativas para enfrentar problemas emocionales como la depresión y la ansiedad. Restaurar el funcionamiento a través de la implementación de un plan de acción y proveer intervenciones adecuadas a las personas con problemas de salud mental es parte de su práctica diaria en las clínicas de salud mental de la comunidad. El enfoque de sus intervenciones es la base de su concentración de lo que sucede en **"el aquí y ahora"** y no en el pasado.

Salud mental, como parte de la salud general de las personas, es un componente del crecimiento humano y por lo tanto, del desarrollo de las naciones. La salud mental no sólo se basa en condiciones subjetivas; también se basa en condiciones objetivas. Una mirada comprensiva a esta afirmación supone una comprensión de la salud mental como un elemento que se inserta en la sociedad. La salud mental está relacionada con el despliegue de diferentes capacidades humanas en diferentes momentos de la vida, las cosas que hacemos ya sean pequeñas o grandes. Se trata de construir y desarrollar vínculos activos que sean transformadores de la realidad, que permitan atender las necesidades personales y el bienestar psíquico, así como de los demás.

Trabajo social es una profesión y disciplina académica que está comprometida a mejorar el bienestar social y emocional de las personas, los cambios y la justicia social. Esta profesión trabaja hacia la investigación y la práctica para mejorar la calidad de vida de las personas, los grupos y la comunidad donde viven. El trabajador social clínico desarrolla intervenciones a través de la investigación, la administración, las organizaciones comunitarias locales, la práctica directa, la prevención y la educación. A menudo, la investigación se centra en áreas como el desarrollo humano, la salud mental, la administración pública, la evaluación de programas y el desarrollo comunitario. Los trabajadores sociales están organizados en grupos profesionales, nacionales, internacionales y locales. Trabajo social es una disciplina interdisciplinaria que incluye teorías de economía, educación, sociología, medicina, la filosofía y antropología (NASW, 2012).

Hablar de salud mental entre los Latinos en Nueva York, es hablar de pobreza, estigma y desigualdad. La situación actual de la salud mental es un indicador importante de las condiciones reales de la mayoría de la población Latina. Esto nos ofrece una visión diferente de lo que significa vivir en la pobreza, la exclusión y la desigualdad que nuestra comunidad atraviesa y que debería ser un componente clave de una estrategia integral contra la pobreza.

¿ Que es Cultura??

El término fue usado primero por el pionero Antropólogo Ingles Edward B. Tyler en su libro, Cultura Primitiva en 1871. Tyler dijo que cultura "es un complejo entero el cual incluye conocimiento, creencias, arte, moral, costumbres y cualquier otra capacidades y hábitos adquiridos por el hombre como miembro de la sociedad." Este no esta limitado a los hombres. Las mujeres también poseen y crean esto. Cultura es un grupo complejo de valores y creencias esenciales que se manifiesta en los símbolos, los mitos, el lenguaje, los comportamientos y constituye un marco de referencia compartido para todo lo que se hace y se piensa en una en el grupo. (Melvine, L. M., 2012).

Subcultura:

Es con frecuencia definida como las creencias, actitudes que separan a los grupos de la amplia cultura. Como nivel de subcultura, está formado de diferentes estatus religiosos y socioeconómicos, inclusive de raza. Los Americanos están bastante familiarizados con las subculturas. Con tan solo pasar un día en la ciudad de New York , se puede experimentar las subculturas de lugares como La pequeña Italia, el Barrio Chino, el Barrio Latino en Harlem. La mayoría de las personas en estos Barrios comparten la cultura nacional de ser Americanos, pero se diferencian de la manera en como se visten, lo que comen, y sus costumbres religiosas (Dresser, W., 2017).

Niveles de Cultura:

Hay tres niveles de cultura (Melvine, L. M, 2012), que son parte de patrones del. comportamiento aprendido y las percepciones. Obviamente es el grupo de tradiciones culturales que distingue a una sociedad especifica. Cuando alguien habla de las personas de las culturas italianas, Latinas, chinas, ellos referimos a al lenguaje común, tradiciones y creencias que separa a estas personas de otros. En la mayoría de los casos. Aquello las personas que comparten una cultura lo hacen porque lo adquirieron al ser criado por sus padres y otros miembros de su familia que lo tienen.

El segundo nivel de cultura que puede ser parte de nuestra identidad es subcultura, la cual es definida como las creencias y actitudes que separan a grupos dentro de la amplia cultura. Como nivel de cultura, subcultura esta formada de diferencias en religión, condición socioeconómica, inclusive raza. Los americanos están familiarizados con las subculturas. Solo basta pasar un día en la ciudad de New York para experimentar las subculturas de los lugares como la pequeña Italia, el barrio Chino, el barrio Latino. Muchas de estas personas de esos barrios comparten la cultura nacional de ser americanos, pero se pueden diferenciar de la manera como se visten, lo que comen y sus diferencias religiosas.

El tercer nivel de cultura consiste cultural universales. Estas son patrones de conductas aprendidas que son compartidas colectivamente por la humanidad. No importa dónde viva la gente en el mundo, ellos comparten los mismos rasgos universales.

Modelos de rasgos humanos culturales :

1. Comunicación con lenguaje verbal consistiendo en un grupo limitado de sonidos y reglas gramaticales para la construcción de palabras.
2. El uso de edad y género para clasificar a las personas (ej. Adolescente, jubilado, hombre, mujer).
3. Clasificación de las personas basado en matrimonio y relaciones descendientes y tener términos de parentesco para referirse a ellos (ej., esposa, esposo, madre, padre, tíos, primos).
4. Criando niños en lugar familiar.
5. Tener división sexual de empleo (ej., trabajo de hombres vs. Trabajo de mujeres).
6. Tener el concepto de privacidad.
7. Tener reglas para regular conducta sexual.
8. Distinción entre buena y mala conducta.
9. Tener adornos corporales.
10. Hacer bromas y jugar juegos.
11. Tener arte.
12. Tener ciertas funciones en la implementación de decisiones comunitarias.

Cultura y sociedad no significan lo mismo. Mientras que culturas son un patrón de conductas aprendidas y preconcepciones, las sociedades son un grupo de personas quienes directa e indirectamente interaccionan entre ellas Tyler, W. B. (1871)., Williams, Raymond; 1958).

Conceptos culturales:

Las actividades diarias del autor con clientes/pacientes y familias que sólo hablan español en New York, donde el idioma dominante es el inglés, muestran una comprensión de la complejidad de la sala de emergencia que es la entrada al sistema hospitalario. Estas experiencias también pueden extenderse a personas y familias de países de diferentes idiomas. Aquellos trabajadores sociales clínicos que no tienen conocimiento del idioma español tienen dificultades para comunicarse con los clientes / pacientes y sus familias. La experiencia del autor en el ámbito hospitalario es extensa, ha ejercido en el Bronx Lebanon Hospital Center, Bronx, Nueva York durante más de dos décadas (1989-2013), y al ser ingresado en un hospital cuando llegó por primera vez a los Estados Unidos y no sabía hablar inglés y fue entrevistado por médicos y enfermeras que no hablaban español y con la ayuda de un traductor que tampoco hablaba bien su idioma. Como resultado de esto, el traductor no le entendió y dió información errónea al médico que lo estaba examinando. Por lo tanto, el autor entiende muy bien los problemas a los que se enfrentan los clientes/pacientes cuando son entrevistados por personas que no hablan su idioma. Según Campinha-Bacote (1998), competencia cultural tiene que ver con el conocimiento cultural, las actitudes, el comportamiento y la inclusión de políticas que entrenan a los profesionales para que puedan desempeñarse en diferentes contextos multiculturales.

A medida que Estados Unidos se transforma en un país diversamente racial, multicultural y étnicamente diverso, los trabajadores sociales clínicos necesitan comprender las diferentes perspectivas étnicas, culturales y valores de las personas a las que brindan sus servicios profesionales. La falta de conocimiento y la comprensión de las diferencias sociales y culturales podrían terminar en consecuencias negativas para las personas de diferentes grupos culturales y étnicos. Se requiere de una intervención adecuada para que los trabajadores sociales clínicos respeten y no juzguen a las personas que necesitan su intervención profesional.

Esto implica el respeto a la creencia sobre los problemas de salud física y salud mental, así como la solución de un problema que es presentado por el cliente/paciente. Competencia cultural en esta área de intervención requiere un conocimiento general de las acciones de asistencia que son comunes en la sociedad. Las instituciones involucradas están separadas culturalmente, lo que podría ser difícil para una intervención adecuada, o podría ser que los servicios que se ofrecen son culturalmente inadecuados o no están disponibles. Los administradores de hospitales y centros comunitarios de salud mental deben desarrollar estrategias para contratar, retener y promover dentro de estas instituciones, equipos de diversos profesionales multiculturales que sean competentes en las áreas donde prestan servicios profesionales. Al hacerlo, los clientes/pacientes podrían comunicarse eficientemente en su idioma y obtener servicios de calidad.

Construir centros comunitarios de salud mental competentes, significa cambiar las percepciones sobre otras culturas o grupos étnicos, ¿cómo se comunican y operan? Esto significa que la estructura, el liderazgo y las actividades de una organización deben reflejar los valores, las perspectivas, el estilo de vida y las prioridades de las personas. Debido a que los cambios sociales están sucediendo rápidamente, las organizaciones deben entender la necesidad de contratar profesionales que sean competentes en la cultura y el origen étnico. Como trabajadores sociales, estamos tomando conciencia de que, si no mejoramos nuestras habilidades y capacidad profesional, estaremos paralizados como organización profesional.

El actual clima político hostil de los Estados Unidos podría causar miedo, ansiedad, depresión y estrés entre la población Latina y otros grupos minoritarios. La intimidación y la hostilidad en las escuelas también podrían causar estrés entre los estudiantes Latinos y de otros grupos minoritarios. La discrepancia salarial junto con el uso de las redes sociales y su complejidad de cómo impactan en la salud mental también es un factor importante. Según algunos expertos en salud mental, el estrés no es la única causa principal de los problemas emocionales, pero puede contribuir a exacerbar la necesidad de que las personas con estas condiciones controlen su salud mental. A pesar de que los trabajadores sociales clínicos tratan este tipo de problemas emocionales, los Latinos, como grupo, tienen menos probabilidades de acceder a los servicios de salud mental, especialmente a los niños y adultos mayores.

El trabajador social clínico debe adaptarse al mundo moderno, la globalización donde las instituciones están teniendo un impacto en las reglas y prácticas unilaterales. El aumento progresivo de consumidores socioculturalmente diferentes, especialmente en hospitales y centros comunitarios de salud mental, constituye un desafío para los trabajadores sociales clínicos. La Asociación Nacional de Trabajadores Sociales (NASW, 2001), define el trabajo social como "una profesión que promueve los cambios sociales, las soluciones a las relaciones humanas y empodera a las personas para mejorar su bienestar social." Mediante la utilización de teorías del comportamiento humano y los sistemas sociales, los trabajadores sociales clínicos intervienen en lugares donde las personas se relacionan con su entorno social (persona y ambiente). Los principios y los derechos humanos son fundamentales para el trabajo social clínico.

La afirmación de un grupo de representantes de trabajo social de todo el mundo afirmó claramente que los elementos que abarca la práctica moderna de esta profesión están interrelacionados dentro del mundo exterior y las experiencias psicológicas internas del individuo. Para entender mejor cómo poder ayudar en estas circunstancias, los trabajadores sociales clínicos deben desarrollar la capacidad de evaluar e intervenir en diferentes lugares con individuos, familias y grupos de personas de diferentes grupos étnicos y culturales. Estas intervenciones deben entenderse dentro el contexto funcional jurídico, las necesidades de servicios para los consumidores, con la base firme contra el racismo y la discriminación. Las fronteras entre países están disminuyendo debido a las presiones económicas, geopolíticas, religiones, guerras, conflictos internos y étnicos que provocan, entre otras cosas, migraciones. Es por eso que la competencia cultural en el trabajo social clínico es una necesidad y expectativa de todos los servicios públicos que refleja el aumento multicultural en una sociedad, país o región diversa donde vivimos (Walker, S., & Beckett, C., 2005).

Ciertos tipos de lenguajes connotativos podrían ser ambivalentes, causando malentendidos que podrían asustar al cliente/paciente, así como a la familia. Debido a esto, el trabajador social clínico, el cliente / paciente y los miembros de la familia podrían terminar en situaciones conflictivas. Es necesario que la comunicación sea clara y adecuada entre el trabajador social clínico y el cliente/familia. Los obstáculos lingüísticos podrían superarse cuando el trabajador social clínico habla el mismo idioma del cliente/paciente y de los miembros de la familia. La comunicación no es fácil, incluso cuando las personas tienen la misma historia de experiencias y valores compartidos o hablan el mismo idioma. Hay situaciones en las que las parejas han estado viviendo durante más de treinta años y todavía tienen malentendidos. Noi es de extrañar, por lo tanto, por tanto, encontrar falta de comunicación entre personas que no se conocen. Lo que se dice podría ser escuchado de una manera diferente por la otra persona o también podría ser malinterpretado.

Lumb, D. (1999), define Competencia cultural como "el grupo de conocimientos y habilidades que el trabajador social y otros profesionales de la salud tienen para poder ser competentes multiculturales con los clientes." Trabajo social clínico se ocupa de diferentes componentes de cultura, que incluyen género, raza, orientación sexual, religión, etc. Green, J. (1999), autor de "*Cultural Awareness in the Human Services,*" estaba seguro cuando dijo que la práctica de la competencia cultural debe tener una base de conocimientos, capacitación profesional e intervenciones adecuadas para poder comprender a personas de diferentes culturas y grupos étnicos. Betancourt, J. R (2001), también mencionó que la cultura es un grupo de creencias aprendidas, valores compartidos, estilos de vida, comunicación, práctica, vestuario y puntos de vista sobre lo que tiene que ver con las funciones y las relaciones sociales.

No todos los que hablan español son iguales, por el contrario, estas personas tienen diferentes historias sociales, valores culturales y religiosos. Los países de población hispanoparlantes son geográficamente diferentes, tienen trajes específicos, formas de hablar, así como mezclas étnicas y culturales. Las personas de América Latina están asociadas con diecinueve países de lengua española, en el Caribe, América Central y del Sur. Los siguientes países son: Cuba, República Dominicana, , Puerto Rico, Costa Rica, El Salvador, Nicaragua, Panamá, Guatemala, Honduras, México, Bolivia, Paraguay, Uruguay, Ecuador, Venezuela, Colombia, Chile, Perú Argentina. La excepción es Brasil, donde el idioma oficial es el portugués.

Cuando el trabajador social clínico es de un país diferente al grupo étnico del cliente/paciente, los malentendidos son comunes. El trabajador social, con desconocimiento del idioma del cliente/paciente debe tener cuidado y evitar hacer suposiciones falsas sobre las expectativas del tratamiento que se le ofrecerá. El trabajador social clínico y el cliente/paciente aportan sus propios patrones sociales y culturales a la experiencia de la entrevista, que deben ser resueltos de inmediato, para poder obtener calidad de los servicios de tratamiento.

Sin el entendimiento de cultura, los trabajadores sociales clínicos contribuyen a la opresión cuando ejercen la profesión con clientes/pacientes de otras culturas. Esta es una práctica poco ética y puede causar mucho daño a los clientes/pacientes. (Sue, D., Arredondo, P., McDavis, R., 1992). Los trabajadores sociales necesitan habilidades para evaluar el sistema de los clientes/pacientes. Si este es ignorado, los trabajadores sociales podrían hacer eco a la presión social al asumir que los clientes/pacientes necesitan cambiar, en vez de trabajar con los cambios sociales (Pinderhughes, E., 1989). Por otro lado, falta de competencia cultural podría también conducir a una compensación excesiva por parte de los trabajadores sociales clínicos; quienes podrían pasar mucho tiempo enfocándose en la cultura o podría excluir conductas disfuncionales (Comas-Diaz, L., 1995).

Raza y etnicidad tienen impacto en las relaciones profesionales y competencia cultural inadecuada trae como consecuencia servicios ineficientes. Davis, L., y Proctor, E. (1989), afirman que muchas personas correlacionan la diferencia del color de la piel con las diferencias en creencias y puntos de vista. Un cliente/paciente con un trabajador social clínico de diferente etnicidad cultural podría asumir que el trabajador social clínico no va a entender su punto de vista del mundo en que vive. Esto disminuye la probabilidad de que el cliente/paciente continue recibiendo servicios. Lo contrario es también cierto. Muchas veces los trabajadores sociales clínicos tienen opiniones negativas de aquellos clientes/pacientes a quienes ellos ven como que tienen diferentes puntos de vista de la de ellos. Esta dinámica es menos común y prejuiciosa (Davis, L., y Proctor, E. (1989).

Obstáculos a la competencia cultural:

Aunque el lenguaje es importante, este no es el único obstáculo. Los obstáculos podrían ser cualquier aspecto de la atención de la salud que contribuya al mal uso de esta. Los obstáculos pueden afectar la calidad de los servicios que se ofrecen y también pueden contribuir a las disparidades raciales y étnicas, que incluyen:

1. Falta de diversidad en los centros de salud.
2. Los hospitales y centros de salud mental están diseñados de manera inadecuada para satisfacer las necesidades de una población diversa de clientes/pacientes.
3. Problemas de comunicación entre los proveedores de atención de la salud mental y los clientes/pacientes de diferentes grupos étnicos, culturales, idiomas, sociales y Religiosos.

Competencia cultural es uno de los principales ingredientes para la eliminación de las diferencias en los centros de salud mental comunitarios, y por esa razón cuando los trabajadores sociales clínicos hablan de problemas psicosociales y de salud mental sin comprender las diferencias culturales durante la interacción con los clientes / pacientes, estos pueden intensificarse. Dicho esto, aquellos hospitales y centros comunitarios de salud mental que respetan y responden a la socio-culturalidad y lingüística de una población diversa, podrían ayudar a la creación de resultados positivos de los servicios de atención de salud física y salud mental. Para el desarrollo de competencia cultural, se requiere examinar preferencias y prejuicios, buscando modelos a seguir y compartir en la mejor manera que sea posible con otras personas que tienen la pasión por competencia cultural. El término competencia multicultural surgió de la publicación en Salud Mental por el psicólogo Paul Pedersen en 1998, al menos una década antes de que el término competencia cultural se hiciera popular.

Según Coon, D. (2000), la mayoría de las definiciones de competencia cultural se comparten con una diversidad de profesionales que son del campo de la salud mental. Según Carter, R. (1999), algunos de los beneficios de desarrollar la competencia cultural en cualquier organización, son:

1. Aumenta el respeto y la comprensión mutua entre los involucrados. Trabajo Social Clínico con Latinos en New York-USA
2. Aumenta la creatividad para resolver problemas a través de nuevas perspectivas, ideas y estrategias.
3. Disminuye las sorpresas no deseadas que pudieran retrasar el progreso en la intervención.
4. Aumenta la confianza y la cooperación del cliente/paciente.
5. Aumenta la participación y la colaboración con otros grupos multiculturales.
6. Ayuda a superar el miedo a cometer errores, a la competencia o al conflicto. Por ejemplo. al entender y aceptar a personas de diferentes culturas, hay más. probabilidades de que estas personas se sientan cómodas.
7. Promueve la inclusión e igualdad de derechos.

Los Latinos en New York tienen acceso limitados a los servicios de salud mental que sean conscientes de las diferencias culturales, creencias, matices lingüísticos o prácticas propias de los Latinoamericanos. Los siguientes factores son:

1. Barreras lingüísticas.
2. Falta de proveedores de salud mental conscientes de las diferencias culturales, creencias, matices lingüísticos y practicas Latinoamericanas.
3. Falta de recursos de salud mental en la comunidad Latinoamericana.
4. Capacidad reducida para identificar los síntomas de los problemas de salud mental debido a la falta de información o comprensión.

Datos estadísticos de Latinos en los Estados Unidos:

La palabra "Latino," define una cultura o grupo étnico y no una categoría racial. Latino, refleja el origen latinoamericano de las personas, pero hay que ser cautelosos y evitar el asumir que todos los Latinos comparten el mismo idioma, ciudadanía, o mismas experiencias. A pesar de las muchas diferencias, los Latinos comparten características culturales e históricas (fueron colonia española).

En 2005, la población Latina era el grupo minoritario más numeroso en los Estados Unidos, compuesto por: 14% de la población total, en comparación con el 13% de los afroamericanos y el 5% de los. asiáticos. Para el próximo 2059, se espera que los Latinos sean casi el 29% de la población. Según la Oficina del Censo de los Estados Unidos (2006) y el Pew Hispanic Center (2015), más del doble que la representación de 2005. El estado de Nueva York es el hogar de más de 3.1 millones de Latinos o el 16% de la población (Pew Hispanic Center, 2015). Los Latinos de descendientes caribeños es el grupo más grande de personas de América Latina (58%), seguido por los de descendientes latinoamericanos (15%), seguidos por (12%) de los descendientes mexicanos y (9%) de América Central.

Según el informe del Pew Hispanic Center (2015), los Latinos son el 25% de la población total del estado de Nueva York; El 38% son blancos, el 23% son afroamericanos y el 14% son de Asia y las islas del Pacífico. La mayoría de los Latinos viven en East Harlem, Nueva York, en **"El Barrio,"** como es referido por los residentes Latinos. Según el censo de 2000, los Latinos eran el 52,1% de la población de East Harlem (Manhattan), seguidos por el 35% de los afroamericanos, los blancos el 7,7%. Entre los Latinos, los puertorriqueños son el grupo más grande en el este de Harlem o el 57.75% de la población, seguido por el 16.9% de los mexicanos y el 7.7% de la República Dominicana. Según el Pew Hispanic Center (2015), la población latina ha crecido un 14% o 2'485,260. Según la Oficina del Contralor de Nueva York (2016), casi uno de cada neoyorquino se identifica como Latino o hispano. Entre 1990 y 2014, la población Latina en el estado de Nueva York ha aumentado un 66%, alcanzando casi 3.7 millones (19%) de la población, y la mayoría de ellos viven en el área metropolitana de la ciudad de Nueva York.

La contribución Latina a los Estados Unidos:

Según la Oficina del Censo de los Estados Unidos (2016), en el Estado de Nueva York, el 83% de los Latinos no hablan inglés en sus hogares. La falta de dominio del inglés es un obstáculo importante para su acceso a los servicios médicos y de salud mental. Lo más importante aún es que aquellos que prefirieron obtener servicios de salud mental en español tenían menos probabilidades de acceder a los servicios de salud mental. En comparación con los Latinos con dominio del inglés, aquellos con conocimientos limitados de inglés tenían 65 años o más, con mayores probabilidades de tener seguro médico, todos los factores contribuyen al riesgo de estrés emocional.

Según la Oficina del Censo de Estados Unidos (2016), de los 60.6 millones de Latinos que más contribución hacen al desarrollo demográfico en Estados Unidos sigue siendo en gran mayoría, mexicanos, puertorriqueños y cubanos, pero la cara de la mayor parte de este país está cambiando. Los números del Censo de los Estados Unidos de 2010 demuestran que los Latinos son más del 16% de la población y su número está creciendo a un 43% en la última década. Los Latinos contribuyeron entre 2000 y 2010 al 56% del aumento de la población total de este país. La recesión financiera golpeó más fuertemente a los latinos con la crisis de la construcción, un importante sector de empleo para este grupo minoritario y solo en 2009, 1,4 millones de Latinos se sumaron a este grupo de pobres que en Estados Unidos está determinado por un salario anual muy por debajo de los $22.000 dólares.

Según la Oficina del Censo de los Estados Unidos (2016), la tasa de pobreza entre los Latinos fue de 23.4% en comparación con los Blancos o 12.4%, los afroamericanos 226.2%, los nativos americanos 27.6%, mientras que los asiáticos eran 12.3%. El nivel de educación de los Latinos es notablemente inferior a la población general, el 23.5% de los Latinos ha completado menos de nueve años de escuela secundaria en comparación con el 6.3% de la población general, el 3% de los blancos y el 5.4% de los afroamericanos. El otro extremo de la educación académica, sólo el 12% de los Latinos se han graduado de una universidad, en comparación con la población general, el 31,1% de los Blancos y el 17%.7% de los afroamericanos. Aunque el ritmo de crecimiento de la población latina ha disminuido en los últimos años, la Oficina de Censo calcula que para el año 2050 habrá unos 100 millones de latinos, esto es casi el 25% de la población general.

¿Qué se considera buena salud para los Latinos?

Según una encuesta realizada con médicos y pacientes Latinos en la ciudad de Nueva York, hay una gran diferencia entre los pacientes Latinos y sus médicos con respecto a lo que estos piensan acerca de tener buena salud. Si bien muchos Latinos piensan que su salud es buena, sus médicos no estuvieron de acuerdo en grandes números (Tallaj, R., M., 2018). Y solo un tercio de los Latinos piensan que no reciben la atención médica que necesitan, mientras que dos tercios de los médicos piensan que los Latinos carecen de barreras persistentes para tener acceso a servicios médicos y de salud mental.

La mayoría de los problemas médicos y de salud mental son desatendidos dentro de la comunidad Latina. El tabaquismo, el asma, la obesidad, la diabetes y la hipertensión arterial, la ansiedad y depresión son algunos de los principales problemas de salud, pero la educación en esta área no es comparable con la gravedad de este problema, y los informes sobre educación para la salud mental no están disponibles en español. Del mismo modo, la salud mental, el abuso de drogas ilegales y el alcoholismo siguen siendo estigmatizados. Un tabú, por lo que tiende a ser tratado deficientemente, o no tratado (Tallaj, R., 2018).

Educación:

El nivel de educación de los Latinos es muy inferior al de la población general. Entre los Latinos adultos en la ciudad de Nueva York, entre las edades de 25 años y más, el 35% no se graduó de la escuela secundaria, en comparación con el 14% entre los Latinos adultos. Un porcentaje más bajo de Latinos en comparación con los no Latinos han completado la universidad, 16% vs. 42% (Oficina del Censo de los Estados Unidos, (2018). Aunque el ritmo de crecimiento de la población latina ha disminuido recientemente, la Oficina del Censo de los Estados Unidos (2018), estima que para el próximo 2030 habrá 74,81 millones de Latinos.

La Oficina del Censo de los Estados Unidos (2018) espera que la población Latina adulta crezca alrededor del 55% en las próximas tres décadas, en comparación con el resto de la población Blanca. La población Latina adulta tiene más probabilidades de ser pobre. 24% de los Latinos adultos (en comparación con el 12% de los Blancos). El mal estado de salud físico y mental parece atribuirse al bajo nivel financiero y al tiempo expuesto a ocupaciones que afectan la salud (construcción, carpintería, agricultura, etc.). Poniéndolos juntos, el acceso a los servicios de salud para esta población es extremadamente limitado (NKI Center for Excellence in Culturally Competent Mental Health, 2011).

Cada año, millones de estadounidenses se ven afectados por problemas de salud mental y los Latinos no son una excepción. La población Latina inmigrante y sus hijos encuentran un número alarmante de factores de riesgo y de problemas emocionales. Además, su condición de minoría limitada y su estado migratorio (indocumentados) podrían limitar su acceso a los servicios de salud que necesitan. Según un informe de Zarate, M., (2013), si bien los problemas de salud mental son el resultado de una combinación de genes y factores ambientales, las circunstancias ambientales también juegan una función importante.

Los hijos de inmigrantes Latinos podrían tener dificultades para vivir con expectativas y demandas de una cultura en su hogar y otra en la escuela. Los niños pueden no ir donde sus padres cada vez que tienen problemas o preocupaciones, pensando que sus padres no entienden lo suficiente la cultura. Mientras que la segunda y tercera generación de inmigrantes enfrenta mayores riesgos de problemas emocionales, muchos inmigrantes Latinos no reciben tratamiento de salud mental sólo cuando su condición es de riesgo. Los inmigrantes Latinos están subrepresentados en el sistema de salud y mental y en el tratamiento de problemas que no requieren hospitalización (NKI Center for Excellence in Culturally Competent Mental Health, 2011). Esto significa que con frecuencia los consultorios médicos no se ocupan de las personas con problemas emocionales o que podrían tener el riesgo de lastimarse a sí mismos o a otros. ¿No es justo que cuando una persona entra en el consultorio de un médico aquejado de un problema emocional (ansiedad/depresión) y la primera pregunta es *"¿tienes seguro médico" ¿trajiste tu tarjeta de seguro"?*

Entre cualquier otro grupo étnico en los Estados Unidos, los Latinos tienen la tasa más alta de no tener seguro médico. La falta de seguro impide el acceso a los servicios médicos y de salud mental. En 2007, el 32% de la población Latina no tenía seguro médico en comparación con la población Blanca no Latina, 10.4% (Pew Research Center, 2009). El índice es más alto para los mexicoamericanos mayores, 37.6% que los puertorriqueños, 20.4%, y los cubanos. El 22% de los menores de 65 años no tiene seguro médico. Los niños son el 29% de los menores de 19 y 8 años que no tienen seguro médico, en comparación con el 11% de los Blancos de la misma edad (NKI Center of Excellence in Culturally Competent Mental Health, 2011). La razón por la falta de seguro médico, según la Oficina del Censo de Estados Unidos (2018), se debe a que los empleadores no ofrecen seguro médico y solo el 44% de los Latinos que tienen seguro médico se debe a la ciudadanía, el nivel de educación y las características del lugar de trabajo.

El nivel de aculturación entre los Latinos en los Estados Unidos podría ser un factor para predecir problemas de salud mental y la evidencia de la aculturación ha sido consistente. Ortega, A. N. (2000), informó la posibilidad de un aumento de los problemas emocionales y el abuso de alcohol y sustancias ilícitas entre los Latinos aculturados y a los no aculturados a los Estados Unidos. La forma de vivir en Estados Unidos impone cambios culturales y estrés en la forma de vivir de los Latinos. Adaptarse a la cultura americana podría debilitar la estructura familiar (familismo), si no existe un sistema familiar sólido y la salud mental de los padres, y sus hijos podrían empeorar (Díaz, C. J., Niño, M., 2019). Según estos autores, los inmigrantes Latinos tienen mejor salud y salud mental que los latinos que nacieron en los Estados Unidos.

La fuerte orientación familiar, también conocida como "familismo," podría contribuir a su ventaja para los inmigrantes. Debido al aumento de monolingües y bilingües entre la población Latina en los Estados Unidos. Es por esto importante que los trabajadores sociales clínicos sean multiculturalmente competentes y sensibles para poder obtener resultados positivos. Es la opinión de este autor que cuando los servicios se ofrecen en el idioma del cliente/paciente sin necesidad de un traductor, los Latinos continúan el tratamiento más tiempo que cuando los servicios no son ofrecidos en el idioma del consumidor. idioma.

La familia, su importancia y sus principales transformaciones socioeconómicas:

No hace mucho tiempo que muchos estadounidenses estuvieron de acuerdo en que la vida familiar estaba compuesta por un grupo de creencias amplias y que estas eran aceptadas como hechos reales. En los Estados Unidos, las familias inmigrantes enfrentan muchos desafíos relacionados con el sustento económico, la vivienda, salud (física y mental) y la educación de sus hijos. Algunos obstáculos son la falta de educación, no poder leer o hablar inglés, la falta de familiaridad con el estilo de vida de los estadounidenses, la dificultad para encontrar un empleo estable o uno que pague lo suficiente para poder mantener a la familia y la dificultad de tener acceso a servicios de salud mental.

Cuando hablamos de inmigrantes familiares Latinos, el padre es el que transmite las fortalezas necesarias para sus hijos, él es el principal ausente, simplemente no está allí en su casa, su casa, con sus hijos, con su familia porque está trabajando muchas horas del día. Desafortunadamente, debido a las muchas razones por las que las familias se separan, a pesar de que tienen vínculos que las unen, hay la migración. La migración es el proceso de separación que es más difícil, porque los miembros de la familia no han roto sus vínculos emocionales, pero estos no se rompen por la distancia, o por una vida mejor, pero *¿qué significa una vida mejor cuando debemos estar separados de nuestros seres queridos? ¿Por qué muchas veces solo hablamos del inmigrante que sufre separándose de su familia, pero ¿qué pasa con el sufrimiento de sus padres, su esposa, sus hijos, la novia, la prometida, sus amigos, sus hermanos, los espacios, sus vestuarios, el barrio, la comida, la contraparte, el sufrimiento de la familia cuando ven a su hijo, amigo irse?* Por diferentes razones, sin rumbo, con solo un objetivo de un sueño que es lo que lo mantiene firme en su decisión de irse, con la decepción de su país o de su ciudad. Con muchas injusticias, con su familia en su corazón y mente, no hay miedo, al menos no debe mencionarse porque se debilitaría.

La inmigración y aculturación pueden ser estresantes, inclusive traumatizante. Con frecuencia la inmigración separa a las personas de sus familias extensas, resultando en una enorme pérdida de apoyo (Heyck, 1994). Las políticas y prácticas de inmigración de los Estados Unidos pueden ser intimidantes, no bienvenidas e incluso violentas (Gutiérrez, L., Yeakley, A., Ortega, R. (2000); esto puede causar miedos generalizados o desconfianza a los servicios sociales. Al llegar a los Estados; los inmigrantes deben adaptarse a la cultura diferente, este término es definido como aculturación. Este proceso implica cambiar las propias prácticas culturales mientras aprendan la nueva cultura y deshacerse de la cultura anterior. Este proceso tiene como resultado el cambio de actitudes, valores y conductas. La inmigración individual y las experiencias de aculturación varían según el país de origen y de las circunstancias individuales, como en el caso de este autor.

Consejos para más servicios de salud mental:

El aumento de los problemas de salud mental en la comunidad Latina, en la ciudad de Nueva York y en Long Island es alarmante. Se ha visto exacerbado por los problemas actuales de atención médica como el Covid-19 (coronavirus). También es alarmante para América Latina, donde los recursos son escasos. Por esta razón, este autor sugiere que el trabajo social clínico en salud mental debe ser ampliado, con énfasis en la educación, promoción y prevención de problemas de salud mental. Los trabajadores sociales clínicos proveen servicios de salud mental a individuos, grupos y familias que tienen problemas de salud mental, a través del diagnóstico y la psicoterapia. También es importante señalar que el contexto familiar actual es más complejo, debido a la forma en que las relaciones matrimoniales se formalizan y se rompen.

El estrés de la aculturación es particularmente difícil para las familias Latinas con padres monolingües y con sus hijos que son bilingües y tienen problemas para adaptarse a la cultura estadounidense. Según un informe de la Asociación Americana de Psicología (2013), titulado "La Psicología de la Inmigración en el Nuevo Siglo," los inmigrantes Latinos y sus hijos viven en mundos diferentes y con frecuencia los padres no saben mucho de lo que hacen sus hijos cuando están fuera de su hogar. Esta situación pone presión en sus hijos para que busquen y salgan de sus problemas y qué consejos pueden darles sus padres. A pesar de que hay un aumento de la necesidad servicios de salud mental entre las familias Latinas, muchas familias no buscan estos servicios debido al estigma que tienen sobre los problemas de salud mental.

La Asociación Americana de Psicología (2013) recomienda que los servicios de salud mental se desarrollen en tres fases:

1. Conocimiento cultural del psicoterapeuta.
2. Actitudes y creencias del psicoterapeuta hacia las diferentes actitudes de los clientes/pacientes.
3. Creencias de clientes/pacientes y comprensión personal, habilidades del psicoterapeuta en intervenciones terapéuticas adecuadas disponibles. Esto incluye ofrecer a los clientes /pacientes, un fácil acceso a recursos tales como traductores y asistente legal, así como facilitar el acceso a diferentes programas comunitarios disponibles en la comunidad.

También es necesaria la intervención interdisciplinaria entre los organismos del sistema de salud mental. Es la opinión de este autor que debe haber una transición de colaboración de servicios sin interrupciones entre hospitales, escuelas y centros comunitarios de salud mental. Al hacerlo, los clientes/pacientes continuarán recibiendo servicios de salud mental sin demoras. El sistema de salud mental también podría ayudar a mejorar la salud mental de las comunidades Latinas al ubicarlas donde existe mayor necesidad de servicios de salud mental. Debe haber campañas de información junto con redes de medios en diferentes idiomas, en lugares donde los Latinos se reúnen; tales como iglesias, clubes sociales (Asociación Americana de Psicología, 2013).

Trabajo social clínico multidisciplinario:

Según Abramson, J., &Mizrahi, T. (1996), Garcés, C. (2018-2019), el razonamiento para la participación y colaboración entre los profesionales de la salud se basa en el reconocimiento de la complejidad de los problemas humanos, el nivel de conocimiento y las habilidades de intervención que se necesitan para obtener resultados positivos. El trabajador social clínico intensifica la efectividad de su intervención que son necesarias para obtener resultados positivos. El trabajador social clínico intensifica la efectividad de su intervención al tener conocimiento de la cultura y la historia del cliente/ paciente. La cultura y las tradiciones son componentes importantes. También es importante que el cliente/paciente y su familia puedan compartir sus tradiciones con el trabajador social clínico durante la entrevista inicial. Una buena pregunta personal podría ser: *¿qué es importante en su cultura que me ayudaría a poder ofrecerle mis servicios?* La respuesta a esta pregunta podría ayudar a evitar malentendidos entre el trabajador social clínico y el cliente/paciente y los miembros de la familia (Garcés, C., 2018-2919).

Problemas de salud mental comunes entre la comunidad Latina en Nueva York:

Los Latinos tienen la misma incidencia de problemas de salud mental en comparación con el resto de la población de Nueva York. Sin embargo, ciertas preocupaciones, experiencias, formas de entenderlas y cómo tratarlas podrían ser diferentes. Sin salud mental no podemos estar sanos. Cualquier parte del cuerpo humano, incluido el cerebro, podría enfermarse. Todos pasamos por diferentes eventos o situaciones que ocasionalmente pueden causar altibajos emocionales. Los problemas de salud mental van más allá de nuestras reacciones emocionales que experimentamos durante el transcurso de la vida. Esto tiene que ver con algunas situaciones o condiciones que podrían cambiar el estilo de vivir, ya que estas podrían complicarse y también podrían crear problemas de relación con otras personas, así como en el entorno laboral y perder el empleo. Sin un tratamiento adecuado, los problemas de salud mental podrían empeorar y dificultar la vida cotidiana de una persona (Alianza Nacional sobre Enfermedades Mentales, 2019).

Síntomas de problemas de salud mental:

1. Ansiedad.
2. Miedo.
3. Irritabilidad.
4. Confusión.
5. Depresión.
6. Preocupación excesiva.
7. Autocritica excesiva
8. Olvido.
9. Preocupación excesiva por el futuro.

Los problemas de salud mental más comunes en la comunidad latina:

1. Esquizofrenia
2. Trastorno de ansiedad general
3. Depresión mayor
4. Trastorno de estrés
5. Trastorno bipolar

Otros problemas asociados con la salud mental con la comunidad latina:

1. Intentos suicidas.
2. Consumo excesivo de drogas ilícitas y alcohol.
3. Violencia doméstica.

Según observaciones del autor, la comunidad Latina en Nueva York muestra una predisposición similar a las condiciones de salud mental, en comparación con el resto de la población. Lamentablemente, hay muchas desigualdades en la salud mental y la calidad del tratamiento. Esta desigualdad expone un alto riesgo para los Latinos de tener un colapso de salud mental o situaciones de crisis y poder ser tratados adecuadamente. En general, los Latinos no buscan tratamiento para su salud mental. Según la Administración de Sustancias y Salud Mental, en 2012, solo el 27% de los Latinos con problemas relacionados con la salud mental buscaron ayuda profesional. En general, las personas en las comunidades Latinas no hablan de sus problemas emocionales. Lamentablemente no hay suficiente información sobre esta cuestión, y no podemos saber lo que nadie nos ha enseñado. Muchos Latinos no buscan tratamientos de salud mental porque no reconocen los síntomas, tienen vergüenza o porque no saben dónde obtener ayuda. Esta falta de información exacerba el estigma ya asociado con los problemas de salud mental. Muchos Latinos no buscan tratamiento de salud mental por temor a ser etiquetados como "locos", "esquizofrénicos," ya que esto podría causarles vergüenza.

El estrés de la aculturación según Dillon, F., y colegas (2013), tiene que ver con el estrés psicológico que experimentan los inmigrantes al responder a los desafíos que encuentran mientras se adaptan a una cultura diferente. Décadas de estudios de investigación han despertado interés sobre el impacto de los problemas de salud mental entre los Latinos en los Estados Unidos, haciendo de esto un determinante frecuente de las desigualdades en los servicios de salud mental. El estrés aculturativo está relacionado con múltiples problemas psicosociales y de salud mental, incluyendo ansiedad, depresión, suicidio, alcohol y abuso de drogas ilegales. A pesar de esto, no hay suficiente comprensión sobre las experiencias que están relacionadas con el estrés aculturativo durante los primeros años de inmigrar a los Estados Unidos.

Los Latinos en Nueva York enfrentan muchos factores que podrían aumentar su riesgo de problemas de salud mental. El estrés podría manifestarse a través de la depresión y la ansiedad, lo que podría conducir al uso y abuso de drogas ilegales y alcohol, y en muchos casos, en el suicidio. El estrés también se manifiesta a través de la inmigración, que es la causa de la angustia emocional, el miedo y para muchos inmigrantes la transición de la reubicación es problemática. Según Insel, T. R. (2005), la investigación sistémica dentro de la trayectoria de moratoria y el posterior seguimiento de los indicadores culturales, sociales y vocacionales del funcionamiento familiar podrían ayudar a los trabajadores sociales clínicos a reconocer problemas, ajustes y a participar en la promoción de intervenciones de salud mental, prevención y tratamiento en cada momento. Debido a la limitada evidencia de estudios, más estudios de investigación es necesario, la investigación ayudaría a evaluar las estrategias de intervención para la promoción de la salud mental en las comunidades Latinas para la prevención de problemas de salud mental que responden a problemas de aculturación.

Las diferencias culturales podrían ser la causa para que los trabajadores sociales clínicos diagnostiquen incorrectamente a sus clientes/pacientes. Por ejemplo: Los Latinos generalmente describen sus síntomas que están relacionados con la depresión con "nerviosismo, fatiga o enfermedad física". Estos síntomas están relacionados con la depresión. Sin embargo, cuando el trabajador social clínico no entiende la cultura del cliente /paciente, esto también podría influir negativamente en el tratamiento y no poder reconocer los síntomas de la depresión. A pesar de que los Latinos prefieren ser tratados por profesionales Latinos de salud mental, desafortunadamente esto no es posible debido al pequeño porcentaje de trabajadores sociales clínicos Latinos bilingües y que sean culturalmente competentes.

Para entender las razones de las disparidades culturales, nos ayudará a construir un sistema de salud mental que pueda combinar la calidad superior de los servicios de salud mental eficientes. Los Latinos conforman un tercio de los ocho millones de habitantes de la ciudad de Nueva York. Pero incluso cuando representamos a una parte sustancial del Estado de Nueva York, y como población en aumento, son invisibles. Son invisibles porque son diferentes, y con estos factores juntos, la atención de la salud física y mental está en crisis. En comparación con los residentes de Nueva York, muchos inmigrantes Latinos carecen de beneficios de atención médica, carecen de atención médica de calidad. Los inmigrantes Latinos enfrentan obstáculos que los hacen más riesgosos de enfermarse (Tallaj, R.M., 2018).

Tanto la presentación de los problemas emocionales como la forma en que son explicados por los Latinos es diferente. Según Lewis-Fernández, E, et al. (2005), los Latinos con problemas emocionales tienen más probabilidades de presentarse con quejas psicosomáticas en comparación con los estadounidenses blancos. Esta podría ser la razón por la que los Latinos tienen menos probabilidades de buscar tratamiento médico para estos problemas, en vez de buscar tratamiento de salud mental. Es importante también entender que la presentación somática de la depresión entre los Latinos podría hacer que los médicos cometan errores, terminando con un diagnóstico incorrecto, exámenes médicos innecesarios y un tratamiento inadecuado (Lewis-Fernández, (et al., 2005).

Los Latinos tienen diferentes maneras de creer acerca de sus problemas emocionales: Muchos Latinos creen en espíritus o pecados por la causa de su enfermedad; una interpretación que hasta la fecha no puede ser entendida por los profesionales de la salud mental. Estas personas pueden utilizar diferentes lenguajes que les impidan reconocer y entender sus problemas. La falta de entendimiento para distinguir adecuadamente los problemas culturales emocionales comunes podría contribuir a la demora en la búsqueda de ayuda para sus problemas, el tratamiento inadecuado y resultados negativos.

Uno de los trastornos culturales conocido entre los Latinos es el *"ataque de nervios,"* el cual es un lenguaje de desesperación que es particularmente común entre los Latinos del Caribe y es también reconocido por muchos Latinos. Esto se describe en los Criterios Diagnósticos del DSM-5 (2013) de los trastornos culturales y los síntomas incluyen: Escalofríos incontrolados, ataques de llanto, temblores corporales, calor en el área del pecho a la cabeza, tornándose verbal o físicamente agresivo. Por lo general, el "ataque de nervios" se produce debido a un evento de estrés, especialmente relacionado con problemas familiares. Con frecuencia, después del "ataque de nervios," es común que la persona sufra amnesia de lo ocurrido, pero poco después vuelve a su funcionamiento normal.

Con frecuencia, el "ataque de nervios" se compara con un episodio de "ataque de pánico" debido a la similitud de los síntomas. Tanto los ataques de pánico como los ataques nerviosos tienen una asociación cerrada con la ausencia de síntomas de miedo y pánico (Guarmaccia, P.J., 2008). Debido a que el ataque de nervios se describe como una reacción emocional temporal a las circunstancias de la vida diaria, la persona no puede reconocer el problema emocional debilitante o la necesidad de buscar servicios profesionales de salud mental (NKI Center for Excellence in Culturally Competent Mental Health, 2009).

Si bien los síntomas de susto son como los del DSM-5 Diagnostic and Statistical Criteria Manual of Mental Health Disorders (2013) de la depresión, las complicaciones para su tratamiento son diferentes. Tradicionalmente, el tratamiento para el susto consiste en una práctica de rituales culturales, con el propósito de llamar al alma a volver al cuerpo para "limpiar" a la persona afectada y devolver el equilibrio total a su cuerpo. Tales rituales son conocidos por el hombre de la medicina tradicional Latina (curandero). Mientras que aquellos clientes/pacientes que sufren de susto pueden experimentar alguna mejora en el tratamiento convencional para los síntomas de la depresión mayor. La falta de entendimiento de las creencias culturales de los clientes/pacientes podría limitar la eficiencia de la intervención terapéutica, afectar la adherencia, y modificar la confianza (o falta de confianza) en el sector de la salud mental formal. El acontecimiento del miedo de los síntomas precipitados podía ser correlativo con el diagnostico diferenciado occidental. Por ejemplo, el miedo debido a un conflicto de una correlación mayor con el diagnóstico diferencial occidental del trastorno de depresión mayor (Guarmaccia, P. J., 2008).

Los desafíos son aún mayores para las personas que solo hablan español. Para ellos al tener que ir a una entrevista con el trabajador social clínico y tener que expresar sus sentimientos/problemas en su propio idioma. La traducción puede ser útil, pero el trabajador social clínico debe tener buena comprensión del contexto cultural para poder ayudar al cliente/ paciente. Dialectos diferentes también podrían complicar la traducción. Muchos inmigrantes Latinos prefieren no buscar ayuda profesional de salud mental o confiar en los trabajadores sociales clínicos debido a la falta de comprensión cultural y competencia profesional para entender sus problemas. Según La Alianza Nacional Sobre Salud Mental (2017), uno de cada cinco Latinos sufre de un problema de salud mental. Los Latinos tienen una orientación colectiva, siendo esta la orientación familiar (familismo), de ayuda mutua y unidos, estos son lazos familiares de la cultura Latina (National Alliance on Mental Health, 2011). Familismo, es una palabra única en el idioma español que enfatiza una fuerte relación familiar (segura), que podría ayudar como un factor protector que promueve el apoyo social que protege a las personas contra los síntomas de la depresión, incluyendo situaciones ambientales de alto riesgo (National Alliance on Mental Health, 2011).

A pesar de que se está reconociendo la depresión mayor en la mujer Latina, el riesgo y los mecanismos de protección que se asocian con los efectos en los niños cuando la madre sufre de depresión, es bien entendido por las familias Latinas. Durante el Censo de 2000, las mujeres Latinas eran el 51% de la población Latina en los Estados Unidos (Bureau of Census de los Estados Unidos, 2000). La mayoría de las mujeres Latinas se concentran en ocupaciones de bajos salarios, trabajan en fábricas, restaurantes, limpieza de casas, peluquerías, recepcionistas, lavanderías, floristerías. Las mujeres Latinas tienen el doble de desempleo en comparación con las mujeres estadounidenses Blancas, y sufren múltiples desventajas sociales y económicas, como el bajo nivel de educación, desempleo, bajos ingresos económicos , madres solteras, los altos niveles de pobreza y víctimas de la violencia doméstica. Estos factores afectan su salud mental y limitan su acceso a los servicios de salud y atención de salud mental. Las mujeres Latinas que nacen en los Estados Unidos tienen un nivel de riesgo más alto de depresión mayor e intentos de suicidio que las mujeres no Latinas (Giachello, A., 2001).

Un estudio de Lewis. M. J. y colegas. (2005), descubrieron niveles significativos de estigma asociados a los síntomas de la depresión y la medicación antidepresiva. Los Latinos que participaron en el estudio recibieron tratamiento para la depresión dijeron que una experiencia con síntomas depresivos se describe negativamente, vista como una característica dentro del contexto social. Cuando las mismas personas fueron entrevistadas sobre las complicaciones que se adhieren a la terapia con medicamentos antidepresivos, el 73% de los participantes hicieron comentarios con referencia al estigma, la medicación antidepresiva, seguidos por el 87% de los efectos secundarios de la medicación. Tener que tomar medicamentos antidepresivos parece ser desaprobado por las familias de los participantes y de su apoyo al sistema social. Los miembros de la familia Latinas también pueden desalentar a sus seres queridos de educación o creencias espirituales o culturales de buscar tratamiento o tomar medicamentos debido a la falta de entendimiento acerca de problemas emocionales.

Servicios de salud mental frente a remedios caseros (Botánica)

El bajo índice de utilización de servicios de salud mental entre la población Latina se atribuye a las consecuencias sociales de buscar estos servicios. El estudio sugiere que los Latinos no buscan ayuda por miedo a la deportación, la desconfianza de los proveedores y el miedo a las autoridades (Lewis, M.J., et al., 2005). Otros estudios sugieren que las personas tienen miedo de avergonzar a la familia cuando buscan servicios de salud mental. Según el mismo estudio, los Latinos ven los problemas emocionales como algo muy privado y no debe ser compartido con otras personas fuera de la familia. Los Latinos pueden estar menos preparados que los estadounidenses Blancos en la búsqueda de servicios de salud mental porque tiene apoyo de su familia. Los recursos sociales incluyen familiares, amigos, padrinos, afiliaciones religiosas, personas espirituales y de otro tipo que practican curaciones y grupos de ayuda personal. Estos recursos se utilizan con frecuencia en lugar de los servicios profesionales de salud mental. Sin embargo, la literatura sugiere que estos recursos no reemplazan efectivamente los servicios profesionales.

Estigma sobre la salud mental entre los Latinos en Nueva York:

Según la Organización Mundial de la Salud (2016), el estigma de la salud mental es la mayor barrera comunitaria para mejorar la salud mental global, y en las culturas Latinoamericanas, este estigma puede ser más frecuente. La OMS (2016), informa que el estigma en torno a la mala salud mental es el mayor obstáculo en el camino de las personas que buscan tratamiento. Estigma se refiere a un conjunto de creencias negativas, y a menudo injustas o inexactas, que la sociedad asocia con ciertas circunstancias, cualidades o personas.

El estigma de la salud mental se refiere a actitudes o creencias negativas que conducen a la "devaluación, deshonra y desfavorecimiento por parte de las personas con enfermedades mentales". Hay tres tipos comúnmente reconocidos de estigma de salud mental (Mascayo, F., Tapia, T., et al., 2016):

1. **Estigma social o público:** Se refiere a las creencias o actitudes discriminatorias negativas sobre las condiciones de salud mental promovidas en el grupo cultural o en la sociedad en general.
2. **Baja autoestima:** Esto ocurre cuando una persona internaliza actitudes sociales negativas sobre las condiciones de salud mental.
3. **Estigma institucional:** Se refiere a las políticas institucionales gubernamentales o privadas que discriminan intencionalmente a las personas con afecciones de salud mental.

El estigma de la salud mental sigue siendo un importante factor negativo que influye en la forma en que las personas tratan y perciben las condiciones de salud mental. El estigma de la salud mental existe en todas partes del mundo, pero puede ser particularmente fuerte en las culturas y comunidades Latinoamericanas (Mascayo, F; Tapia, T., et al., 2016).

Estigmas comúnmente indican que las personas con problemas de salud mental son:

1. Violentos, agresivos o con dificultad de actuar fuera de lo común.
2. Incapaces de mejorar.
3. Peligrosos y debe ser aislados o mantenidos alejados del público.
4. No pueden realizar las mismas actividades o deberes que otros.

Algunos elementos de la cultura o sociedad Latinoamericana que pueden influir en cómo se establece, percibe e impacta el estigma de la salud mental:

1. **Familismo:**

Es un termino que se usa para describir fuertes conexiones familiares, que involucra sentido de lealtad y obediencia (Gelman, C., 2004). La familia incluye la familia nuclear, familia extensa, amigos, vecinos que están fuertemente vinculados a la familia. Dentro de las familias, existen funciones que son típicas de las madres, padres y los hijos. Machismo es un termino utilizado para describir la creencia de que los hombres son los proveedores y es su obligación mantener a las familias seguras (Comas-Diaz, L., 1995). "Marianismo" describe a las mujeres como espiritualmente superiores a los hombres y por la tanto, capaces de soportar grandes sufrimientos, mientras que "hembrismo" describe la fuerza y perseverancia de las mujeres. El grado de machismo y de marianismo presente en las familias según Anderson, S., y Sabatelli. (1995), es variable. Estas funciones influyen en la dinámica familiar y necesitan ser considerados durante las intervenciones clínicas. [por ejemplo, las mujeres puertorriqueñas pueden mostrar marianismo en el hogar y hembrismo en el lugar de empleo; este entendimiento puede ayudar a los trabajadores sociales clínicos para entender una aparente conducta contradictorias (Comas-Diaz, L., 1995).

El valor cultural del familismo, o el valor colectivo de la unidad familiar, puede desempeñar(Anderson, S., Sabatelli, R. (1999). una función en la formación y aplicación del estigma de la salud mental entre los Latinos (National Alliance on Mental Health, 2011). Este valor puede estar asociado con el aumento de las tasas de actitudes hostiles de la familia y la familia extendida, así como los miembros de la familia que subestiman las habilidades de alguien. Al enterarse del diagnóstico psiquiátrico, las familias a menudo experimentaron frustración, negación y dolor (Uribe, R., et al., 2007). Hablar de problemas de salud mental entre familiares es considerado como un tabú. Esto significa que evitan hablar de este tema entre familiares y amigos.

2. Religión:

El culto religioso y las actividades de la iglesia son parte de socialización cultural Latina. La espiritualidad es importante para los Latinos y es un recurso de apoyo emocional (Gelman, C., 2004). Mientras que la mayoría de Los latinos son católicos, no podemos asumir que todas las familias son católicas o devotos. Algunos Latinos creen en espíritus (curanderismo). Los clientes/pacientes Latinos pueden buscar tratamiento por medio de la medicina de los curanderos al mismo tiempo que reciben tratamiento médico y de salud mental (Comas-Diaz, L., 1995).

La fe también parece jugar una función importante en la conformación del estigma que los Latinos pueden tener sobre los problemas de salud mental. Los Latinos tienden a depender de las instituciones religiosas como un importante recurso espiritual, educativo y social. Según un estudio de 2019 que exploró las creencias sobre las condiciones de salud mental en las comunidades Latinas basadas en la fe en Nueva York. Las creencias religiosas pueden contribuir a los estigmas al hacer cumplir los conceptos erróneos de que:

1. La mala salud mental es una falla moral o un dilema espiritual.
2. La mala salud mental es una condición espiritual, más que médica.
3. La mala salud mental es un castigo o una forma de justicia divina.
4. La depresión se debe a la falta de fe, a no orar lo suficiente, a comportamientos pecaminosos hacia los padres u otros, o a la influencia demoníaca. Orar y tener fe en Dios puede ayudar a reducir el riesgo de o tratar las afecciones de salud mental.
5. Los actos autolesivos, como el corte o el suicidio, se deben a la falta de fe verdadera.

Los latinos que viven en Nueva York también pueden tener un acceso reducido a la atención de salud mental adecuada debido a los siguientes factores:

1. Barreras lingüísticas.
2. Falta de proveedores de atención de salud mental conscientes de las diferencias culturales, creencias, matices lingüísticos o prácticas Latinoamericanas.
3. Falta de recursos sanitarios especializados en la comunidad.
4. Una capacidad reducida para identificar los síntomas de la enfermedad mental debido a la falta de información o comprensión.
5. Estatus legal personal o estatus legal de un ser querido.

Para reducir el estigma que rodea a la enfermedad mental, la Alianza Nacional Sobre Enfermedades Mentales (2011), recomendó lo siguiente:

1. Hablar abiertamente de salud mental.
2. Educarse a sí mismo y a los demás sobre la salud mental.
3. Promover la idea de que la mala salud física y mental son lo mismo.
4. Ser consciente del lenguaje que puede ser estigmatizante, como los términos "loco", o "psicótico".
5. Informar a los medios de comunicación cuando están promoviendo el estigma negativo.
6. Mostrar compasión a las personas con afecciones de salud mental.

Botánicas (tiendas étnicas de remedios caseros), se encuentran particularmente en la ciudad de Nueva York. Las botánicas son tiendas que ofrecen remedios caseros religiosos, productos espirituales y servicios a un cliente diverso que son en su mayoría de América Latina y los países del Caribe. La presencia de botánicas en la ciudad de Nueva York está relacionada con la presencia de dispensarios (farmacias que aparecieron en 1900). Estas botánicas están en áreas donde los Latinos son la mayoría. Además, las botánicas ofrecen servicios de asesoramiento a las personas que buscan orientación espiritual y emocional en una variedad de situaciones, desde problemas financieros hasta emocionales (asesoramiento). La percepción de la efectividad de la práctica en el hogar, combinada con las hierbas medicinales que se ofrecen en las botánicas son baratas (bajo costo), y de fácil acceso, atraen a los Latinos que buscan servicios informales de salud mental (Gómez, A., Beloz, J., et al ., 2011).

En un estudio reciente de Pérez Porto, M. (2017-2019), los curanderos dijeron ser capaces de curar una amplia variedad de sufrimientos fisiológicos, espirituales y emocionales. También dijeron tener una forma única de diagnosticar y curar, en comparación con el modelo de los Estados Unidos: las causas psicosomáticas que son el resultado de la demanda social. Los Latinos con problemas físicos y emocionales tienen la tendencia a hacer menos uso de los servicios de salud mental que los estadounidenses blancos. En 2007, sólo el 26,6% de los Latinos con problemas de salud mental recibieron servicios, en comparación con el 50% de los Latinos blancos. Los latinos mayores en necesidad de servicios de salud mental tienen menos probabilidad de tener acceso a los servicios de salud mental que los latinos no Blancos y cuando los reciben, estos tienen mas probabilidad de ser de mala calidad (Institute of Medicine (IOMD0, 2003). United states Department of Health and Human Services (USDHHS0).

Uso personal profesional:

La práctica del trabajo social clínico con Latinos exige una cuidadosa evaluación personal y comprensión de cómo los trabajadores sociales ven el mundo que los rodea y cómo la sociedad dominante afecta su intervención profesional con los Latinos. Por lo tanto, los trabajadores sociales clínicos deben ser conscientes de su propio sesgo y de cómo su visión del mundo afecta su concepto de clientes / pacientes. Por ejemplo, si el punto de vista de un trabajador social clínico es valorar el individualismo, él / ella debe evaluar críticamente cómo dirigirse a un cliente / paciente desde un punto de vista colectivo (Furman, R., y colegas., 2006).

Los Latinos valoran las relaciones personales íntimas. También valoran la función del clínico para adoptar una "tradición médica/paciente", especialmente al inicio de la relación profesional. También es importante entender por qué a los Latinos les gusta saber la vida personal del clínico. Como trabajadores sociales, clínicos debemos entender que esto no es una cuestión de límites profesionales.

El desarrollo de una fuerte relación terapéutica es crucial. Personalismo se refiere a los valores que los Latinos ponen en las relaciones interpersonales. Los trabajadores sociales clínicos que no son Latinos deben de ser sensitivos a este tema y adaptar su estilo de expectativas de los clientes/pacientes Latinos. Algunas de las modificaciones podrían incluir la cantidad de información personal, aceptar regalos (con frecuencia comida) y mas contacto físico (saludo con las manos, palmadas en la espalda, llamar por el primer nombre), así como también la cercanía del espacio (Gelman, C., 2004). Además, las intervenciones deben tener enfoque a la solución, directa y activa (Gelman, C., 2004). Debido a que los Latinos valoran respeto, los trabajadores sociales clínicos deben entender la jerarquía y poder dentro del sistema familiar. Es también importante desarrollar relaciones personales antes de proceder con la relación profesional (Gutiérrez y colegas., 2000). Parte de este proceso implica que los trabajadores sociales clínicos y clientes/pacientes aprendan de mutuamente de sus sistemas de creencias. Las disparidades en los sistemas de creencias deben de ser mencionados, de esta manera ellos pueden empezar el tratamiento con entendimiento mutuo (Yeh, M., y colegas., 2004).

Trabajadores sociales en salud mental:

Debido al éxodo de los trabajadores sociales de los hospitales, estos tuvieron que encontrar nuevas funciones para sí mismos. Decidieron entrar en áreas de salud mental y hacerse útiles en este campo. Esta inclusión en salud mental tiene una historia (Instituto Nacional de Salud Mental, 1991). Desde hospitales de psiquiatría hasta el desarrollo de centros comunitarios de salud mental, los trabajadores sociales se han encontrado proporcionando psicoterapia a individuos, grupos y familias. Además, los trabajadores sociales han estado activos en la prevención real de las enfermedades mentales causadas por eventos mundiales actuales como el Covid-19. Se están haciendo esfuerzos para desarrollar programas públicos y asignar fondos, para asegurarse de que las enfermedades mentales se traten con el mismo grado de gravedad que otras enfermedades médicas.

Al trabajar con otros profesionales de la salud mental (psicólogos, psiquiatras), los trabajadores sociales comenzaron a colaborar en el desarrollo de teorías de la etiología y de intervenciones, que ahora se han probado a través de la práctica y la investigación. Sin embargo, sin ser un investigador desprevenido, el énfasis en la salud mental en lugar del entorno social ha cambiado el curso histórico del trabajador social típico. En lugar del individuo y su entorno (persona y ambiente), el trabajador social clínico busca justificar la práctica por los mismos motivos que el médico, que suscribe el enfoque biopsicosocial para el consumidor. Esto puede parecer un pequeño detalle en una gran vista panorámica del lugar del trabajador social clínico en la sociedad, pero no es un pequeño zancudo que vuela en el ambiente. Ahora los trabajadores sociales clínicos trabajan en la psique del individuo, ayudándole a encontrar la felicidad, la paz dentro de sí mismo y a mejorar su salud mental. El entorno social de los consumidores se ha quedado en la atención histórica del problema.

El objetivo principal de los trabajadores sociales clínicos en salud mental es poder ayudar a las personas que sufren de trastornos emocionales, para que puedan funcionar en el mundo en el que viven. Esta nueva función adoptada ha ayudado a mejorar las condiciones de los enfermos mentales, que ya no están encerrados en instituciones psiquiátricas. El concepto suscrito ahora de ser el trabajador social clínico ayuda al consumidor a "adaptarse" a las realidades de la vida (Instituto Nacional de Salud Mental, 1991).

A diferencia de los psiquiatras y psicólogos, los trabajadores sociales clínicos están capacitados para tener interés en toda la persona. Sin embargo, estas funciones y entornos adoptados son desafiantes, ya que el modelo médico es difícil de apartar. Prevalece, y esto significa que la capacitación del trabajador social clínico para tratar a toda la persona choca de frente con el enfoque de la psiquiatría, que es curar la enfermedad emocional mediante la prescripción de medicamentos psicotrópicos (Instituto Nacional de Salud Mental, 1991). Lo que esto realmente significa es que incluso la función adoptada por el trabajador social clínico, ser el defensor de los enfermos mentales también ha sido desafiado. El trabajador social clínico típico en un hospital psiquiátrico o una clínica de salud mental comunitaria tiene las manos atadas al psiquiatra que puede no creer realmente que la psicoterapia realizada por un trabajador social clínico ayuda al paciente, tanto como un medicamento antipsicótico. Si esto es cierto, podría haber sido más sabio para el trabajador social clínico permanecer en el entorno hospitalario, donde convertirse en un huérfano para ser adoptado no era una opción.

La experiencia profesional de este autor en salud mental comunitaria comenzó después de graduarse de Fordham University en 1985. Fue en el Puerto Rican Family Institute en el Sur del Bronx, Nueva York, donde ejerció por primera vez como trabajador social psiquiátrico. La población del sur del Bronx era principalmente puertorriqueña, de la República Dominicana y de otros países de América Latina. Posteriormente, en 1997 pasó a trabajar en el Queens Neuropsychiatric Institute en Jackson Heights Queens, Nueva York donde la mayoría de los clientes/pacientes son de Perú, Chile, Argentina, Ecuador, Bolivia, México, Colombia, Uruguay, Venezuela. Desde 2010 ha estado ejerciendo como psicoterapeuta en Community Counseling Services en Long Island, Nueva York, donde los clientes / pacientes son mixtos; Estadounidenses y latinos, en su mayoría de Honduras, El Salvador, Guatemala, México.

Según un informe de la Organización Mundial de la Salud (OMS-2013), la salud mental se define como un estado de bienestar en el que un individuo es consciente de sus propias capacidades, es capaz de enfrentar los factores estresantes de la vida normal, puede trabajar productivamente y capaz de contribuir a la comunidad. La dimensión positiva de la salud mental se destaca en la definición de salud que figura en la Constitución de la Organización Mundial de la Salud (2013): La salud es un estado de completo bienestar físico, mental y social, y no sólo sobre la ausencia de afectos o enfermedad. La salud mental incluye nuestro bienestar emocional, psicológico y social. Afecta la forma en que pensamos, sentimos y nos comportamos cuando enfrentamos problemas desafiantes. También ayuda a determinar cómo manejamos el estrés emocional, cómo nos relacionamos con otras personas y cómo tomamos decisiones. La salud mental es importante en todas las fases de nuestra vida desde el nacimiento hasta el final de la vida.

Comprensión del trabajo social clínico:

Trabajo social clínico es una especialidad del trabajo social médico, que se ocupa del asesoramiento, la psicoterapia y la coordinación de servicios (planificación del alta) a personas con problemas de salud mental, y en algunas situaciones necesitan hospitalización psiquiátrica u otro tratamiento psiquiátrico. Los trabajadores sociales clínicos tienen una variedad de tareas al tratar a clientes/pacientes, incluyendo pero no limitado a evaluaciones psicosociales, psicoterapia individual, familiar y de grupo, intervención de crisis, apoyo emocional y coordinación de atención médica y planificación de alta. Los trabajadores sociales pueden ejercer en diferentes instituciones: Hospitales, sistema judicial, escuelas, drogas y centros de rehabilitación, centros del oficio de enfermera y de la rehabilitación, centros de salud mental de la comunidad.

Los trabajadores sociales clínicos pueden trabajar como:

1. Administradores de clínicas de salud mental
2. Investigadores.
3. Hospitales psiquiátricos y médicos.`
4. Administradores de casos (abuso y negligencia infantil, violencia doméstica, abuso de ancianos).
5. Psicoterapeuta.

El trabajo social clínico es una especialidad que cumple con los siguientes requisitos:

1. Tiene un cuerpo sistémico de teorías que apoya lo que hace.
2. Tiene autoridad profesional que emana del dominio de la teoría.
3. Tiene conocimiento comunitario de que la profesión es válida.
4. Tiene un código de ética que rige la conducta de sus miembros, tiene una cultura profesional dentro de un vocabulario, y una metodología profesional.

El trabajo social clínico basa su metodología en el campo sistémico de la evidencia basada en el conocimiento derivado de la investigación y la evaluación práctica, incluyendo sus propios conocimientos y un contenido específico. También reconoce las interacciones complejas entre las personas y su entorno, y la capacidad de los individuos para reaccionar cuando se ven afectados por múltiples influencias o circunstancias sobre sí mismos, incluidos factores psicosociales, de salud y ambientales como el COVID-19. La profesión de trabajo social extrae de las teorías del desarrollo humano, la teoría social y la teoría de sistemas sociales para analizar situaciones complejas y familiarizar los cambios individuales de las organizaciones culturales y sociales .

Los trabajadores sociales clínicos proveen servicios de salud mental (psicoterapia) a individuos, familias y grupos de individuos que tienen problemas emocionales. Los trabajadores sociales clínicos proveen psicoterapia y diagnostican problemas emocionales mediante el uso del DSM-5 Diagnostic and Statistical Manual of Mental Disorders (2013). La función del trabajador social clínico varía según el lugar de la práctica. En el ámbito hospitalario es sobre todo la planificación del alta. Esto comienza tan pronto como el paciente es admitido en el hospital y tiene lugar al momento del alta del paciente del hospital. A veces, los pacientes necesitan servicios especiales como referencias a hogares de ancianos de enfermería y rehabilitación, rehabilitación ortopédica, rehabilitación de drogas y alcohol (Garcés, C., 2018-2019). Durante la planificación del alta, el trabajador social clínico debe asegurarse de que el paciente tenga todos los recursos necesarios antes de regresar a casa y poder funcionar en la comunidad. Actualmente, la estancia hospitalaria es más corta que hace unos años (Garcés, C., 2018-2019., NASW, 2007).

Actualmente, los trabajadores sociales clínicos laboran en hospitales psiquiátricos, clínicas de salud mental de la comunidad. Entre otras misiones de trabajo social psiquiátrico en el campo de la psiquiatría hay:

1. La prevención de problemas emocionales a través de la detección anticipada de casos susceptibles.
2. La explicación a los usuarios de los servicios de salud mental.
3. Implementación de mediciones para mejorar el tratamiento de seguimiento como, por ejemplo, organización de grupos familiares, autoayuda, colaboración en campañas de concientización sobre salud mental.

El trabajador social clínico:

Es un profesional capacitado para evaluar y generar cambios en la persona que acude a su consultorio para consulta y psicoterapia, el cual se da con el propósito de mejorar la calidad de vida a través de cambios en el comportamiento y las actitudes. El trabajador social psiquiátrico hace uso del Manual Diagnóstico y Estadístico de Salud Mental FDS-5 (2013), para la evaluación de problemas emocionales. El trabajador social psiquiátrico es un trabajador social clínico con licencia, que ayuda a las personas a mejorar sus vidas, a desarrollar mejores habilidades cognitivas y emocionales, reducir los síntomas de angustia emocional para poder enfrentar adversidades. Este profesional es una persona que ayuda a las personas a recordar que son valorados y apreciados por los demás.

El trabajador social clínico como psicoterapeuta familiar:

1. Educa a los miembros de la familia sobre el papel de la familia como grupo, particularmente, cómo funcionan entre ellos.
2. Ayuda a la familia a centrarse menos en el miembro que fue identificado como "problemático" y a centrarse más en la familia como unidad.
3. Ayuda a identificar conflictos y ansiedades, así como a trabajar juntos para desarrollar estrategias para resolverlos.
4. Fortalece a todos los miembros de la familia para que puedan trabajar juntos para resolver problemas.
5. Enseña maneras de resolver problemas y cambios dentro de la familia. A veces, la forma en que los miembros de la familia resuelven sus problemas hace que tengan más probabilidades de desarrollar síntomas depresivos.

Modelos de práctica de trabajo social clínico (NASW, 2014):

1. **Resolución de problemas. El** enfoque de este modelo es la comprensión del problema, la búsqueda de diferentes ideas para resolver el problema, permitiendo al cliente / paciente encontrar una solución, probar la solución, y más tarde, evaluar el resultado de la solución.
2. **Concentrarse en la tarea.** El enfoque de este modelo es separar el problema en pequeñas áreas que el cliente /paciente puede lograr. El trabajador social clínico puede usar esto como una práctica, límite de fecha y contrato, para ayudar al cliente / paciente a poder sentirse exitoso y motivado para resolver problemas
3. **Concentrarse en la solución.** El enfoque de este modelo es comenzar con la solución, más tarde ayudar al cliente/paciente a establecer pasos para llegar a la solución del problema.
4. **Terapia narrativa.** El enfoque de este modelo está en el uso de palabras y otros modelos para ayudar al cliente / paciente a empoderar su vida.
5. **Psicoterapia cognitiva (CPT).** Este modelo combina la psicoterapia cognitiva con la psicoterapia conductual, identificando patrones inadecuados del proceso de pensamiento y respuestas emocionales o conductuales, sustituyéndolas por patrones deseables de pensamiento, respuestas emocionales o comportamiento. ¿Cómo controlar la ansiedad y el estrés? Aprender técnicas de relajación como, respiración profunda, hablar en voz alta, decir: "Hice esto antes", y distracciones, identificar situaciones que con frecuencia se pueden evitar y poco a poco acercarse a situaciones de miedo.

Los atributos que son característicos del trabajo social clínico incluyen la perspectiva del uso del respeto por parte de la persona en el ambiente, por la importancia de los derechos de los clientes/pacientes, y una fuerte alianza terapéutica entre el cliente/paciente y el trabajador social clínico. Con más de 200,000 trabajadores sociales clínicos que atienden a millones de clientes/pacientes, los trabajadores sociales clínicos constituyen un gran grupo de proveedores de servicios de salud mental en los Estados Unidos (Center for Clinical Social Work, 2007-NASW, 2014).

La base de conocimientos del trabajo social clínico incluye teorías de la biología, el desarrollo psicológico y sociológico, la diversidad y la competencia cultural, las relaciones interpersonales, la dinámica familiar y grupal, los trastornos de salud mental, las adicciones, el impacto de la enfermedad, los traumas o lesiones, los efectos físicos, el entorno social y cultural. Estos conocimientos se inculcan en las escuelas de posgrado de trabajo social y se integran en las habilidades de práctica directa que son desarrolladas por el estudiante durante aproximadamente dos años de experiencia de posgrado bajo la supervisión de un trabajador social clínico (CSW). Este período es suficiente para preparar al trabajador social clínico para poder ejercer de forma independiente con una licencia del Estado como trabajador social clínico profesional. En los años siguientes, los trabajadores sociales clínicos pueden obtener una práctica más generalizada o pueden decidir especializarse en una o más áreas de la práctica.

El trabajo social clínico es importante debido a las habilidades de sus practicantes para poder adaptarse a diferentes entornos y funciones, incluyendo el jefe de los miembros del equipo en centros multidisciplinarios y en centros comunitarios de salud mental. Clientes/pacientes, individuos, parejas, familias, niños y grupos, se benefician de una amplia variedad de servicios directos que incluyen, entre otros, evaluaciones psicosociales, planes de tratamiento, intervención en crisis y manejo de casos. La aplicación hábil y flexible de conocimientos, teorías y métodos de intervención con el enfoque psicosocial, es un sello de calidad del trabajo social clínico.

El proceso directo de intervenciones, se llevan a cabo con personas de todas las edades y de diferencias naturales, desde servicios de prevención, intervenciones de crisis, psicoeducativas, hasta la defensa de los derechos de los clientes/pacientes, así como el extenso proceso de psicoterapia. Muy a menudo, los trabajadores sociales clínicos supervisan y consultan con otros colegas y también pueden participar en la práctica directa e indirecta (administración, investigación, escritura). Es un estándar de práctica para que los trabajadores sociales clínicos continúen la educación clínica y se adhieran al código de ética profesional (Center for Clinical Social Work Research, 2007).

Trabajo social en el centro hospitalario:

trabajo social fue introducido a los hospitales en los Estados Unidos por el Dr. Richard Cabot en 1905. El Dr. Cabot creó la primera posición de trabajo social en el mundo, dándosela primero a Garmet Pelton, y más tarde fue seguida por Ida Cannon (Davidson, K., 1998). En 1918, se estableció la Asociación Nacional de Trabajadores Sociales (NASW), con el propósito de mejorar la relación entre la educación formal y la práctica en los hospitales. El papel de los trabajadores sociales era proporcionar servicios sociales a las personas necesitadas, sin embargo, los administradores sólo querían que los trabajadores sociales evaluaran las necesidades sociales de los pacientes para aliviar a los médicos y evitar el abuso del hospital por parte de los pacientes (Davidson, K., 1990).

El *trabajador social en el centro hospitalario:*

1. Comunica: enfatiza la comunicación entre el personal médico, los pacientes y sus familias, y se asegura de que se satisfagan sus necesidades médicas.
2. Ofrece apoyo emocional: centrándose en cuestiones psicosociales y las necesidades emocionales de los pacientes y sus familias.
3. Defensores: por los derechos del paciente asegurándose de que el hospital brinde servicios médicos de calidad.
4. Enlaces: asegurarse de que los recursos disponibles para los pacientes son adecuados.
5. Consejo: personalizar las interacciones y comprender los sentimientos, actitudes y comportamientos de los pacientes y sus familias.
6. Interviene: entre pacientes, familiares y personal médico.
7. **Coordina:** organización de servicios para pacientes tras su alta hospitalaria.
8. Educa: transmitir el conocimiento y enseñar sobre los derechos de los pacientes, incluidas las decisiones médicas y los problemas del final de la vida.

Según el autor, los trabajadores sociales hacen poco o nada para promocionarse a sí mismos y sus servicios clínicos. Las habilidades y contribuciones no son evidentes para los propios trabajadores sociales clínicos. Por ejemplo, el trabajador social puede no saber que se necesitan habilidades para estar en una habitación con un paciente que sufre a pesar de que el trabajador social ha recibido años de capacitación. Todos los años de formación educativa, sin embargo, van al borde del camino cuando el trabajador social clínico es cuestionado acerca de sus habilidades en este ejemplo. Esto es extraño; porque los médicos y enfermeras saben cuáles son sus habilidades en este caso. Como señalan Davidson (1990) y Cowles, L. A., 2000, el trabajo social hospitalario ha desarrollado una fuente de conocimiento y ha influido en la atención al paciente al promover el reconocimiento del componente psicosocial de la atención de la salud. Los trabajadores sociales en entornos de atención médica llevan un modelo de atención centrada en la persona y la familia a la evaluación y el tratamiento, que difiere del modelo médico centrado en el paciente (Garcés, C., 2019).

La experiencia de este autor como trabajador social clínico en el entorno hospitalario comenzó en 1989 en el Bronx Lebanon Hospital Center en el Sur del Bronx, Nueva York, el cual es uno de los barrios más pobres de los Estados Unidos y está compuesto por personas de casi todo el mundo. Además, la gente del sur del Bronx sufre de múltiples problemas médicos, asma, diabetes, sida, colesterol, hipertensión, obesidad. También hay problemas psicosociales y de salud mental. Delincuencia, el uso indebido de drogas y alcohol, la prostitución, la falta de vivienda, el abuso de niños y ancianos y la violencia doméstica. Según el informe de la Oficina del Censo de los Estados Unidos (2006), más del 38% de la población del sur del Bronx vive por debajo del nivel de pobreza. Las cifras son peores para los niños: el 49% vive en la pobreza (Bronx Lebanon Hospital Center, 2007).

Los trabajadores sociales laboran en hospitales, educando al personal médico sobre la planificación del alta, las intervenciones de crisis, los cuidados paliativos, uniendo a los pacientes y a las familias con los recursos comunitarios disponibles. Los trabajadores sociales clínicos colaboran con médicos y enfermeras y otro personal médico (Mizrahi, T., Abramson, J., 1985., Garcés, C., 2002), para identificar las necesidades sociales de los pacientes, no sólo el problema actual. Si bien el tiempo de las visitas domiciliarias es parte del pasado, los trabajadores sociales clínicos continúan participando en las evaluaciones de las situaciones familiares, reforzando los apoyos sociales que están disponibles para aquellos pacientes que están dados de alta del hospital y que necesitan continuar con la atención Garcés, C., 2002-2019). El trabajador social clínico contribuye a la operación general del entorno hospitalario ayudando / ayudando a los pacientes y sus familias a hacer frente a la crisis, incluida la muerte y con el proceso de planificación del alta del hospital.

El/la trabajador social en el hospital también:

1. Evalúa los problemas social-ambientales de los pacientes
2. Ayuda a los pacientes a examinar posibles soluciones a sus problemas socioeconómicos
3. Ayuda/asiste a pacientes de recursos comunitarios para sus problemas social- ambientales
4. Contactar a las agencias comunitarias para solicitar servicios para sus problemas social-ambientales de los pacientes
5. Informar a los pacientes de cómo sus problemas médicos pueden crear problemas social-ambientales para ellos
6. Refiere a pacientes al personal apropiado del hospital para la ayuda con sus problemas social-ambientales

Durante la pandemia del Covid-19, los trabajadores sociales clínicos han estado desempeñando sus funciones clínicas con el proceso de alta fuera del hospital, en sus hogares. Los médicos y las enfermeras requieren un contacto directo con los pacientes en los hospitales. Debido a la pandemia, los hospitales tuvieron que reducir la cantidad de personal que se consideraba "esencial", entre ellos estaban los trabajadores sociales. Estas regulaciones fueron impuestas por los gobiernos federales y locales. Los trabajadores sociales clínicos no pudieron comunicarse directamente con los pacientes con Covid-19 y sus familias debido a este mandato. La planificación del alta se proporciona a través de una sesión de telesalud con pacientes y familias.

El/la trabajador social clínico es un profesional que tiene una maestría o doctorado en trabajo social de una escuela acreditada de trabajo social. Además de al menos dos años de experiencia supervisada post-maestría en un entorno clínico. El/la trabajador social debe tener licencia, certificarse o estar registrado a nivel clínico en la jurisdicción de la práctica. Un trabajador social clínico proporciona servicios directos, incluyendo dinámicas intrapsíquicas, y problemas de manejo de la vida. Los servicios de trabajo social clínico se basan en perspectivas biopsicosociales. Los servicios consisten en diagnóstico, tratamiento (incluyendo psicoterapia y asesoramiento), intercesora centrada en el cliente, consulta, evaluación y prevención de enfermedades mentales, trastornos emocionales o conductuales.

Los trabajadores sociales pueden trabajar como:

1. Administradores en clínicas comunitarias de salud mental.
2. Investigadores.
3. Rehabilitadores.
4. En hospitales médicos y psiquiátricos.
5. Gestores de casos.
6. Psicoterapeutas.
7. Catedráticos.

Trabajo social clínico es una especialidad que cumple con los siguientes requisitos:

1. Tiene un cuerpo sistemático de teorías que sostiene su trabajo.
2. Tiene autoridad profesional que emana del dominio de la teoría.
3. Tiene reconocimiento comunitario de que la profesión es válida.
4. Tiene un código de ética que rige el comportamiento de sus miembros.
5. Tiene una cultura profesional consistente y vocabulario y metodología profesional.

Trabajo social clínico basa su metodología en el conocimiento derivado de la investigación y la evaluación de la práctica, incluyendo sus propios conocimientos con un contenido específico. Asimismo, reconoce la complejidad de las interacciones entre las personas y su entorno, y la capacidad de las personas para reaccionar ante múltiples influencias o circunstancias sobre sí mismas, incluyendo la salud psicosocial o factores ambientales como el Covid-19. Ttrabajo social extrae de las teorías del desarrollo humano, las teorías sociales y de sistemas para analizar situaciones complejas para familiarizarse con los cambios individuales dentro de las organizaciones sociales y culturales (NASW-Definition of Social Work, 2000).

El/la trabajador social clínico como psicoterapeuta familiar:

1. Enseña a todos los miembros de la familia acerca de cómo funciona la familia en general, y cómo funcionan ellos mismos.
2. Ayuda a la familia a centrarse menos en el miembro que fue identificado como "problemático" y a centrarse más en la familia.
3. Ayuda a identificar conflictos y ansiedades, también ayuda a la familia a desarrollar estrategias para resolverlos.
4. Fortalece a todos los miembros para que puedan trabajar juntos en la solución de sus problemas.
5. Enseña maneras de resolver conflictos y cambios dentro de la familia. A veces, la forma en que los miembros resuelven sus problemas hace que tengan más probabilidades de desarrollar síntomas depresivos.

La base de conocimientos del trabajo social clínico incluye las teorías de la biología, el desarrollo psicológico y sociológico, la diversidad y la competencia cultural, las relaciones interpersonales, la dinámica familiar y grupal, los problemas emocionales, las adicciones, el impacto de los problemas emocionales en las personas, los traumas. Estos conocimientos se fomentan en las Escuelas de Graduados de Trabajo Social y se integran en las habilidades de práctica directa que son desarrolladas por los estudiantes durante aproximadamente dos años de experiencia de posgrado bajo la supervisión de un trabajador social clínico. Este período de capacitación es suficiente para preparar al trabajador social clínico para poder ejercer de manera autónoma con licencia del Estado como trabajador social clínico. En los años siguientes después de la graduación, los trabajadores sociales clínicos pueden obtener una práctica avanzada generalizada o pueden también decidir especializarse en una o más áreas.

Trabajo social clínico es importante debido a las habilidades de sus practicantes para adaptarse a diferentes funciones, incluidos jefes de departamento en centros multidisciplinarios, en hospitales (médicos/ psiquiátricos) y en centros comunitarios de salud mental. Los clientes/pacientes, los individuos, las parejas, las familias, los niños mayores y los grupos se benefician de una amplia variedad de servicios directos que son proporcionados por los trabajadores sociales clínicos, incluidas las evaluaciones psicosociales, el tratamiento, la intervención en crisis y el manejo de casos. La aplicación hábil de conocimientos, teorías y métodos de intervención, con el enfoque biopsicosocial, es un sello de calidad del trabajo social clínico.

Las intervenciones de proceso directo de persona/personas, se realizan con personas de casi todas las edades y diferentes por naturaleza, desde servicios preventivos, intervención en crisis y servicios psicoeducativos hasta la defensa de los derechos de los pacientes, así como el corto o extenso proceso de asesoramiento y psicoterapia. Por lo general, los trabajadores sociales clínicos supervisan y consultan con otros colegas y también pueden participar en la práctica directa e indirecta (administración, investigación, escritura). Esta es una norma de práctica para que los trabajadores sociales clínicos participen y continúen una larga y extensa carrera para continuar su educación clínica y adherirse al código de ética profesional (Center for Clinical Social Work Research, 2014).

La profesión de trabajo social ha evolucionado de la filantropía y la teoría del bienestar a la tecnología social, en términos recientes, es considerada como una disciplina científica en el desarrollo de las ciencias sociales, que guía una profesión con un espacio definido en la satisfacción de las necesidades humanas, existencialmente (material) y apreciativamente (afectivo y político). El trabajo social clínico se reinventa y tiene sentido con respecto a una visión holística de su realidad (NASW, 2014). Con la llegada de la globalización de los mercados financieros, el avance científico y tecnológico, los trabajadores sociales clínicos deberían estar pensando desde una dimensión más integral e interdisciplinaria, con nuevos métodos de intervención, donde podamos mejorar el bienestar y el bienestar de las personas, las familias y la sociedad.

Trabajo social no clínico:

El trabajador social no clínico puede incorporar psicoterapia en organizaciones públicas o privadas, y en la gestión de casos. Muchas veces, los trabajadores sociales no clínicos pueden trabajar brindando asesoramiento y ayudando a los clientes a encontrar empleo, coordinar programas de rehabilitación, prevención de programas de abuso infantil / abuso y negligencia de ancianos. Por lo general, esta práctica hace que trabajen con clientes basados en consultas (NASW, 2014).

Un trabajador social clínico ¿Es lo mismo que un consejero/psicólogo?

Cuando las personas hablan de psicoterapia, por lo general se refieren a este término a psicoterapeuta, trabajador social clínico, psicólogo, consejero en el contexto de trabajar con las personas para mejorar sus problemas de salud mental. Estos términos tienen el mismo significado y se pueden intercambiar. El uso del término sobre otros es solamente sobre la preferencia. El consejero y el asesoramiento son más comunes que la psicoterapia y el psicoterapeuta en los Estados Unidos (NASW, 2014).

Con frecuencia, los trabajadores sociales clínicos y los psicólogos tienen las mismas funciones. Los trabajadores sociales clínicos pueden atender los problemas emocionales, de conducta o emocionales de clientes/pacientes. Los trabajadores sociales clínicos no hacen uso de las evaluaciones psicológicas para dar un diagnóstico. Los trabajadores sociales clínicos no necesitan tener doctorado estudian la conducta humana y pueden diagnosticar y tratar problemas de salud mental, ellos utilizan evaluaciones psicológicas para el diagnóstico. Ambos, psicólogos y trabajadores sociales clínicos tienen como propósito de ayudar a clientes/pacientes con sus problemas a través de la evaluación y tratamiento. Los psicólogos necesitan el doctorado mientras que los trabajadores sociales clínicos no.

Una lista de diferentes términos que los latinos en Nueva York usan como sinónimo de psicoterapia:

1. Consejero.
2. Consejero de salud mental.
3. Psicólogo.

Psicoterapeuta, el significado es el mismo, pero la gente lo refiere a la terapia, esta es una versión corta, y tiene mejor uso que la psicoterapia. El término es útil porque puede referirse a un terapeuta de masaje, u otra clase de profesional.

¿Cómo se diagnostican los problemas psiquiátricos?

De acuerdo con la referencia de escritorio a los criterios de diagnóstico (DSM-5 (2013):

1. Es necesario un historial médico del cliente/paciente.
2. Examen físico y trabajo de laboratorio.
3. Evaluación psiquiátrica, psicológica o psicosocial, que tiene preguntas sobre pensamientos, sentimientos y comportamiento.

Ideas equivocadas sobre lo que se entiende por trabajador social clínico / psicoterapeuta:

Para entender mejor lo que significa un psicoterapeuta, primero debemos hablar de lo que no lo es. Hay muchas ideas y conceptos erróneos sobre el significado de psicoterapeuta. Aquí algunos de ellos:

1. **Ideas equivocadas: El trabajador social clínico / psicoterapeuta es como un amigo a quien la gente paga para escuchar:**
   Para pensar que el trabajador social clínico / psicoterapeuta es un amigo que es contratado, descuente la cantidad de educación y capacitación profesional que se requiere para mejorar la salud mental de las personas a las que servimos. La mayoría de los trabajadores sociales clínicos/psicoterapeutas tienen seis años de educación. Otros tienen más de una década de estudios profesionales.

2. **Ideas equivocadas: El trabajador social/psicoterapeuta clínico le dice a la gente qué hacer:**
   La mayoría de los trabajadores sociales clínicos/psicoterapeutas no le dicen a nadie lo que deben hacer. No hay como sus padres, maestros o entrenadores. No dictan ni gritan instrucciones a seguir. Los trabajadores sociales clínicos /psicoterapeutas trabajan con personas a las que enseñan habilidades para poder vivir una vida saludable y ser capaces de tomar buenas decisiones. Los trabajadores sociales clínicos/psicoterapeutas empoderan a las personas y tratan de no crear dependencia.

3. **Ideas equivocadas: El trabajador social clínico / psicoterapeuta, lee la mente:**
   El trabajador social clínico/psicoterapeuta no trata de adivinar lo que el cliente/paciente está pensando o analiza sus ideas. La principal preocupación del trabajador social clínico/ psicoterapeuta está en lo que el cliente / paciente está pensando, sólo porque quiere ayudar.

Cinco teorías que describen la práctica clínica del trabajo social (Engard, B., 2017).

1. **Teoría Psicosocial.** Su enfoque está en la forma en que las personas son moldeadas y cómo reaccionan a su entorno.
2. **Teoría Psicodinámica.** Trata de entender el comportamiento de las personas.
3. **Teoría Transpersonal.** Fue influenciado por Carl Jung, utiliza influencias positivas, en lugar de enfermedades humanas, y defensas para la realización del potencial humano. Esta teoría utiliza santos, artistas, héroes y otras figuras similares. Las personas que tienen un buen ego pueden tratar de emular como modelos a seguir y aspiraciones.
4. **Teoría cognitiva del aprendizaje.** Su enfoque está en los efectos del medio ambiente, y refuerza el comportamiento, sin embargo, Bandura, A (1977) añadió dos dimensiones importantes: Las fuerzas de mediación siguen entre el estímulo y la respuesta, y las personas pueden aprender el comportamiento a través de la observación.
5. **Teoría de sistemas.** Afirma que el comportamiento está influenciado por una variedad de factores que trabajan juntos como un sistema. Los padres, los amigos, la escuela, el estatus social, el entorno del hogar y otros factores influyen en la forma en que una persona piensa y se comporta.

Guías para la intervención con personas con trastornos de salud mental:

1. Ser respetuoso.
2. Estar tranquilo, claro y directo en la comunicación.
3. Ser consistente y predecible.
4. Establecer límites, reglas y expectativas.
5. Mantener la distancia profesional
6. Aceptar al cliente/paciente tal y como es.
7. Atribuir síntomas a la enfermedad.
8. No tomar los síntomas de la enfermedad como personales.
9. Mantener una actitud positiva incluso durante el fracaso
10. Reconocer y alabar el comportamiento positivo.
11. Ayudar al cliente a establecer metas y objetivos realistas.
12. Tener la actitud de "no sé" ante las preguntas difíciles.

Valores éticos:

Según la Asociación Nacional de Trabajadores Sociales (NASW, 2002), el código de ética son normas de comportamiento moral para una sociedad o grupo, como los trabajadores sociales. El código de ética para una profesión tiene estándares de comportamiento para una determinada profesión. Estos códigos éticos reflejan preocupaciones y definen principios básicos que ayudan como orientación profesional. Su finalidad es:

1. Provee una posición práctica para ayudar a los profesionales en la toma de decisiones hacia los clientes / pacientes y la sociedad.
   a. Garantiza a la sociedad que los profesionales van a demostrar sensibilidad con respecto a las expectativas sociales.
   b. Garantiza a los profesionales el respeto de su integridad y libertad.
   c. Ayuda a aclarar las responsabilidades que los profesionales tienen hacia los clientes/ pacientes.
2. Los trabajadores sociales deben evaluar la práctica ética en las siguientes **consideraciones:**
   a. El juicio moral profesional (no incomodar al cliente/paciente).
   b. Aspectos legales (leyes que rigen).
   c. Implicaciones éticas (aplicar principios éticos que deben ser respetados).
3. Este código de ética se divide en cinco secciones:
   a. El objetivo principal es ayudar a las personas necesitadas y centrarse en sus problemas.
   b. Justicia social; desafiando la injusticia social.
   c. Dignidad y valentía de la persona. Respeto por el individuo.
   d. Importancia de las relaciones humanas.
   e. Integridad: práctica dentro del área de especialización y compromiso con mejores habilidades profesionales.

Recordar y considerar:

1. Las necesidades de los clientes/pacientes.
2. Nivel de competencia profesional del trabajador social clínico.
3. Orientación clínica del trabajador social clínico.
4. Competencia cultural del trabajador social clínico con el cliente/paciente.
5. Los trabajadores sociales clínicos deben respetar el código de ética profesional.

Requisitos para el éxito en trabajo social clínico:

1. **Eliminar la barrera del idioma:** La comunicación es esencial para diagnosticar problemas de salud mental, por lo que comprender lo que expresan los clientes / pacientes es
2. fundamental. El uso de intérpretes puede ayudar, pero un trabajador social clínico que habla el idioma nativo del cliente / paciente, y puede entender los matices culturales y la jerga, a menudo es eficaz.
3. **Colaboración con médicos de atención primaria:** Colaborar con los médicos de atención primaria es importante para llegar a la población Latina.
4. **Fomentar la participación familiar:** Los latinos tienen un sólido sistema de apoyo familiar. El apoyo familiar puede aliviar el estigma de los problemas de salud mental y alienta a los clientes para abordarlo. Compartir información con los miembros de la familia aumenta su comprensión del problema y les ayuda al cliente/paciente.
5. **Proporcionar un tratamiento sensible y culturalmente competente:** Una intervención adecuada con clientes / pacientes que solo hablan español requiere una comprensión de ambos idiomas, también requiere las habilidades para comunicarse de manera eficiente en cualquiera de los dos idiomas en diferentes niveles. Los problemas en la evaluación de los problemas de salud mental del cliente / paciente podrían ocurrir cuando hay una falta de comprensión de los contenidos étnicos, culturales, sociales y económicos que son importantes para la comprensión de las actitudes sobre las necesidades sociales y el comportamiento. La dificultad para hacer evaluaciones también puede ocurrir cuando el trabajador social clínico no tiene la capacitación adecuada para las intervenciones en salud mental.
6. **Educar sobre las razones fisiológicas de los trastornos emocionales:** La falta de información y los malentendidos exacerbarían el estigma. Informar detalles sobre el diagnóstico psiquiátrico, discutir los planes de tratamiento y responder preguntas podría ser la mejor manera de eliminar el estigma. Explicar las causas biológicas y ambientales de las enfermedades mentales es educativo para muchos Latinos.
7. **Empatía:** Es la habilidad de identificar y entender los puntos de vista de las experiencias e otras personas (NASW, 2003). Ponerse en "los zapatos" y reconocer sus experiencias, percepciones y puntos de vista que permite a los trabajadores sociales clínicos entender y desarrollar fuertes relaciones con sus clientes/pacientes. Esta es una habilidad vital que ayuda a los trabajadores sociales clínicos identificar las necesidades de los clientes/

pacientes, basado en sus experiencias únicas para lograr servicios eficientes (Barker, R.L., 2003).

8. **Comunicación:** (verval-nonverbal), esta es una vital habilidad de los trabajadores sociales. La habilidad de comunicarse claramente con una variedad de personas es esencial. los trabajadores sociales clínicos también deben tener buena comunicación con colegas, otros profesionales y deben documentar claramente y reportar información pertinente.

9. **Organización:** Los trabajadores sociales tienen horarios bastante ocupados con responsabilidades de servir y apoyar a clientes/pacientes, incluyendo documentación, reportes escritos y colaboración con otros profesionales. Esto requiere que los trabajadores sociales clínicos deben ser organizados y capaces de priorizar las necesidades de los clientes/pacientes para mantener en orden sus casos. Desorganización y mala organización puede ser causa de que los trabajadores sociales clínicos no proveen atención adecuada a las necesidades de los clientes/pacientes y resultar en consecuencias negativas.

10. **Pensamiento crítico:** Es la habilidad de analizar información y obtener información sin tener preferencias inclinadas de observación y comunicación. Trabajadores sociales deben tener la habilidad de evaluar cada caso colectando información a través de información, entrevistas e investigación. El pensar críticamente y sin prejuicios y haciendo decisiones, identificando, haciendo uso de recursos y formulando las intervenciones mas adecuadas para los clientes/pacientes.

11. **Escuchar cuidadosamente:** Escuchar cuidadosamente es necesario para que los trabajadores sociales clínicos entiendan las necesidades de los clientes/pacientes. Escuchar cuidadosamente, concentrándose, hacer preguntas adecuadas, utilizando técnicas tales como, parafraseando y resumiendo para ayudar al desarrollo de confianza con los clientes/pacientes.

12. **Atención personal:** Trabajo social clínico puede demandar estrés emocional. Es por eso importante en participar en actividades que ayuden a mantener una vida balanceada. La atención personal se refiere a las prácticas que ayuden a reducir el estrés y mejorar el bienestar personal, fatiga, y esto es crucial para una profesión sostenible. Al prestar atención a la persona, los trabajadores sociales clínicos, estarán entrenados a proveer servicios profesionales a sus clientes/pacientes.

13. **Competencia cultural:** Ejercer la práctica de trabajo social clínico con clientes/pacientes de diversos grupos étnicos y culturales, requiere respeto y responder a las creencias culturales y políticas de otras personas. Los trabajadores sociales deben tener conocimiento y respeto por las historias culturales, examinar su historia cultural mientras que buscan conocimientos necesarios, habilidades y valores que puedan mejorar la provisión de servicios profesionales a las personas de diferentes experiencias culturales que están asociadas con raza, edad, etnicidad, educación, clase social, orientación sexual, religión, o discapacidad física o mental. (NASW, 2003). Al poseer actitud crítica y aprecio por diversidad y valores que puedan ofrecer servicios de calidad a los clientes/pacientes.

14. **Paciencia:** Los trabajadores sociales clínicos encuentran varios individuos y circunstancias en su práctica diaria. Es importante tener paciencia con los clientes/pacientes para poder

intervenir adecuadamente con casos complejos y con clientes/pacientes quienes necesitan prolongados periodos de tiempo para superar sus problemas. Esto les da a los trabajadores sociales clínicos poder para para entender la condición de os clientes/pacientes y así evitar decisiones complicadas y frustraciones que puedan causar errores costosos y resultados negativos para los clientes/pacientes.

15. **Compromiso profesional:** Ser trabajador social clínico exitoso requiere un periodo extenso de aprendizaje. Los trabajadores sociales clínicos deben tener compromiso con los valores, ética y desarrollar competencia profesional. Este compromiso es necesario para lograr la misión de trabajo social, "mejorar el desarrollo humano y ayudar lograr las necesidades de todas las personas, en particular atención a las necesidades de empoderamiento a los mas vulnerables, opresados y viviendo en la pobreza.

16. **Defensor:** Los trabajadores sociales promueven justicia social y empoderan a clientes/pacientes a través de apoyo. La habilidad de apoyar permite que los trabajadores sociales clínicos representen y argumenten por sus clientes/pacientes y los conecten con recursos y oportunidades que son necesarios, especialmente aquellos que son vulnerables o no pueden abogar por sí mismos.

Conclusión y recomendaciones:

Trabajo social es una profesión que está avanzando de una manera que los gobiernos y los empleadores de todo el mundo están reconociendo el tremendo impacto que los trabajadores sociales clínicos tienen con las personas a las que sirven en sus comunidades. Menos delincuencia, mejores resultados en el sistema médico y de salud mental, más personas que tienen acceso al empleo y la educación son el resultado del trabajo social, apoyando a las personas para que tengan el control de su propio futuro y hagan realidad sus aspiraciones. Como profesión basada en los derechos humanos, trabajo social tiene una función esencial en la sociedad abogando por que las comunidades levanten sus voces y defiendan sus derechos junto con los demás. La fuerza de la profesión radica en su capacidad para construir una democracia participativa, unir a las comunidades en un futuro sostenible y defender los derechos humanos.

Durante más de un siglo, trabajo social se ha desarrollado y reinventado en respuesta a los cambios sociales, políticos y económicos, manteniendo su enfoque en la defensa de los derechos sostenibles de los segmentos más vulnerables de la sociedad y el mejoramiento de sude la sociedad y el mejoramiento de su bienestar emocional. Los trabajadores sociales clínicos constituyen el mayor un número de profesionales que laboran en el sistema hospitalario, clínicas de salud mental comunitarias, sistema de educación, sistema judicial, en centros de rehabilitación física, centros de rehabilitación de drogas y alcoholismo, en centros para ancianos, centros de servicios sociales (National Association of Social Workers, (NASW, 2002).

Los trabajadores sociales clínicos tienen una función importante, por lo tanto, elevando las voces de las personas cuyas preocupaciones no siempre se escuchan proporcionalmente. Las personas fuera de la profesión de trabajo social tienen la posibilidad de no estar familiarizadas o informadas sobre los servicios psicoterapéuticos que como trabajador social clínico proporcionan. Falta de conocimiento y comprensión de lo que hacen los trabajadores sociales clínicos en el ámbito hospitalario y en los centros comunitarios de salud mental, podría crear conflictos en la colaboración con otros profesionales en la prestación de servicios. La intervención eficiente de los trabajadores sociales clínicos depende, en parte, de cómo otros profesionales de la salud y el público perciben el papel del trabajador social clínico. El trabajo social clínico moderno debe adaptarse al mundo globalizado, donde las instituciones están impactando las reglas unilaterales y su práctica. El aumento progresivo de los diferentes consumidores socioculturales, especialmente en hospitales y centros comunitarios de salud mental, constituye un desafío para los trabajadores sociales clínicos.

Los trabajadores sociales clínicos ayudan a las personas a recibir atención de calidad que son recursos necesarios para vivir una vida de calidad. Ayudar a los niños con necesidades especiales en las escuelas, ayudar a las personas con enfermedades terminales, con cambios en su vida cotidiana, y proporcionar los servicios de psicoterapia necesarios a las personas con problemas emocionales. Como trabajadores sociales clínicos contribuimos en la sociedad de muchas maneras. Si bien es un requisito el uso de técnicas para ayudar a las personas con diversos problemas médicos, psicológicos y psicosociales, como trabajadores sociales clínicos podríamos beneficiarnos haciendo uso del enfoque holístico.

La ansiedad y la depresión en todo el mundo han aumentado debido a la pandemia de Covid-19 (Coronavirus), que ha traído miedo e incertidumbre entre la población. Para las personas con problemas de salud mental, existe el riesgo de un aumento de estas condiciones. Ahora que algunos lugares han estado abriéndose al público (centros comerciales, restaurantes, tiendas, etc.), la gente está volviendo a su "forma de vida normal". Sin embargo, aquellas personas con problemas emocionales podrían enfrentar serios problemas de adaptación. ¿Cómo podrían pasar por los desafíos de continuar su vida diaria? ¿Cómo podrían ayudarles la familia y los amigos? como trabajadores sociales clínicos? ¿Cómo podríamos ayudarles?

El estigma en torno a la salud mental existe en todo el mundo. Sin embargo, según las limitadas investigaciones disponibles, este estigma puede ser especialmente fuerte en los países y comunidades de América Latina. Es el consejo de este autor que las personas afectadas por el estigma de la salud mental, ya sea directa o indirectamente, pueden considerar abordar esto con sus seres queridos y buscar ayuda de profesionales de la salud mental culturalmente competentes. Ayudar a los latinos a superar su estigma sobre las enfermedades mentales no es fácil. Cuanto más entiendan los trabajadores sociales clínicos la cultura latina, mejor.

El desafío para los trabajadores sociales clínicos es poder demostrar sus habilidades profesionales y clínicas, para poder mejorar el bienestar emocional y social de las personas a las que sirven. Los trabajadores sociales clínicos deben contribuir a las iniciativas de investigación, no sólo para poder demostrar nuestra eficiencia en las intervenciones psicoterapéuticas, sino también para promover el conocimiento y la comprensión entre otros colegas sobre la importancia de identificar y comunicar las necesidades psicosociales y de salud mental de las personas que reciben servicios profesionales. Además, los trabajadores sociales clínicos deben entender que juegan un papel importante al identificar el estrés traumático y las relaciones emocionales cuando diagnostican a una persona con una enfermedad mental y el estigma que aparece. Como clínicos, los trabajadores sociales juegan un papel importante porque son los que dan forma a la sensibilidad cultural de cualquier programa de prevención en su vida profesional. Por lo tanto, las creencias de los valores de los trabajadores sociales, la visión del mundo y las formas de conocimiento son componentes esenciales en los esfuerzos por proporcionar servicios que sean auténticos y culturalmente sensibles. Competencia cultural es actualmente un requisito fundamental para los profesionales de salud mental que ejercen con clientes/pacientes que son culturalmente diversos. Adiestramiento y educación en competencia cultural podría mejorar la calidad de atención de salud mental a los grupos étnicos y culturales.

A manera que los Estados Unidos se convierten en un país racial, multicultural y étnico, los trabajadores social clínicos tienen que entender las diferentes perspectivas étnicas, culturales y valores de quienes proporcionan sus servicios profesionales. Falta de conocimiento y entendimiento de las diferencias sociales y culturales podría tener consecuencias negativas. Las necesidades y demandas para los servicios de salud mental van a aumentar a manera que la población aumenta. Sin los esfuerzos para entender como los Latinos afrontan los problemas de salud mental y cómo poder ofrecerles servicios de salud mental de calidad. Los Latinos seguirán sufriendo desproporcionadamente las necesidades insatisfechas de salud mental (Vega, WA, López, SR (2001). Trabajo social continúa buscando crecer dentro de la jerarquía profesional de manera que pueda también gozar del prestigio, autoridad y monopolio que actualmente pertenecen a otras profesiones consideradas destacadas como, medicina, psiquiatría, psicología.

Datos Estadísticos

Población	Idioma, educación y Pobreza
US Censo 200: Los Latinos eran el 52.1% de la población del Este de Harlem, New York en el Barrio" como es referido por los residentes Latinos.	**Bureau del Censo (2016))**, en el Estado de New York: 83% de Latinos no Habla Español en sus hogares.
Datos estadísticos de Latinos en los Estados unidos (2005): 145 de la población total del Estado de New York.	**El 23% de Latinos** a completado menos de nueve años de educación secundaria, comparada con el 6.3% de la población general, 3% Blancos y 5.4% de Afroamericanos.
Reporte del Pew Hispanic Center (2015): 25% Latinos de la población total del Estado de New York.	**Educacion académica:** Solo el 12% de Latinos se han graduado de la universidad, comparados con la población general, 31.1% de Blancos y 17% de Afroamericanos.
La Oficina del Censo de los Estados Unidos (2018): espera que la población adulta Latina aumente al 55% en las próximas tres décadas, comparada con el resto de la población Blanca. Se estima que para el próximo 2030 habrán 74.81 millones de Latinos en los Estados Unidos.	**Latinos adultos en la ciudad de New York** entre las edades de 25 y más: 35% no se graduó de la escuela secundaria, comparada con el 14% entre los Latinos adultos.
Oficina del Controlador de New York (2016): Casi uno de cada Neoyorquino se identifica como Latino o Hispano. Entre 1990 y 2014 la población Latina en New York aumento a=un 66%, alcanzando casi 3.7 millones (19%) de la población y la mayoría de ellos vive en el área metropolitana de la ciudad de New york.	**Nivel de pobreza: era del 23%.**4 comparada con la población Blanca o 12.4% de Afroamericanos 26.2%, mientras que los Asiáticos fueron el 12.3%.

Bibliografía

Abramson, J. S., Mizrahi, T. (1996). Cuando los trabajadores sociales y los médicos colaboran: Experiencias interdisciplinarias positivas y negativas. Journal of the National Association of Social Workers, (4), 2-28.

Anderson, S. y Sabatelli, R. (1999). Family interaction: A multigenerational developmental perspective. (2nd ed.). Needham Heights, MAS: Allyn & Bacon.

Asociación Americana de Psicología (1979-1988). ¿Qué es la Psicoterapia? In Bloch Sidney (Ed). An Introduction to the Psychotherapist. Oxford University Press, p. 92-92.

Comas-Diaz, L. (1995). Puerto Ricans and sexual child abuse. In L.A. Fontes (Ed.), Sexual abuse in nine North American Cultures: treatment and prevention (pp.31-66). Thousand Oaks, CA: Sage Publications.

Oficina del Censo de los Estados Unidos. American Fact Finder-Results. Factfinder.census. gov. Consultado el 16 de enero de 2020.

Bandura, A. (1997). Teoría del Aprendizaje Social. New York General Learning Press. Betancourt, J. R. (2001). Competencia Cultural. ¿Movimiento marginal o dominante? New England Journal of Medicine; 351: 953-955.

Campinha-Bacote, J. (1998). A Model and Instrument for Addressing Cultural Competence in Health Care. Revista de Educación en Enfermería; 38 (5), 204-207. Google Académico.

Carter, R. (Ed), (1999). Abordar los problemas culturales en las organizaciones. Más allá del contexto corporativo. Thousand Oaks, CA: Sage Publications.

Centro de Trabajo Social Clínico. (2007). ¿Cuál es la diferencia entre el trabajo social clínico y no clínico? Junta Americana de Examinadores en Trabajo Social Clínico.

Coon, D. (2001). Introducción a la Psicología. Puertas de entrada a la mente y el comportamiento. Novena edición. Warthworth.

Davis, L., & Proctor, E. (1989). Race as an issue in practice. In race, gender & class: Guidelines for practice e with individuals, families, and groups (pp.1-19). Englewood Cliffs, NJ: Prentice Hall, Inc.

Davidson, K. (1990). Desenfoque de roles y la búsqueda del trabajador social para un dominio claro. Salud y Trabajo Social, 15, 228-234.

Desk reference To the Diagnostic Criteria From DSM-5. (2013). American Psychiatric Association Publishing. Washington DC, Londres-Inglaterra.

Christina, J. J., Niño, Michael. (2019). Familism and the Hispanic Health Advantage: The role of Immigrants status. Sage Journals.

Dillon, F. R., De La Rosa, G. E., Ibáñez, J. (2013). Estrés aculturativo y disminución de la cohesión familiar entre los inmigrantes latinos. Springer.

Engard, Brian. (2017). 5 Teorías de Trabajo Social que informan la práctica. Ayudante de Trabajo Social.

Fernández, R. L., Das, Amar, K., Weissman, César Alfonso Myrna. (2005-2011). Depression in US Hispanics: Diagnostic and Management Considerations in Family Practice. The Journal of The American Board of Family Practice, 18 (4), 282-296.

Gelman, C. (2004). Empirically based principles for culturally competent practice with Latinos. Journal of Ethic & Cultural Diversity

Garcés, C.M. (2002). El trabajador social en la sala de emergencias. Tesis Doctoral. Universidad de Yeshiva (WWSSW). Nueva York., 13 (1), 83-108.

Garcés, C.M. (2018). La Intervención del Trabajador Social en el Centro Hospitalario-Retos para la Profesión. Edición Revisada. Palibrio Publishing Company.

Garcés, C.M. (2019). Intervenciones de Trabajo Social Hospitalario. Gold Touch Publisher.

Guarnaccia, P. J. (2008). Ataques de pánico en la población latina: ¿Culturalmente ligados y distintos de los ataques de pánico?

Gutierres, L., Yeakley, A., Ortega, R. (2000). Educating students for Social Work with Latinos: Issues for the new millennium. Journal of Social Work Education, 36, 541-557.

Giachello, A. (1999). Hispanic Health Rx. University of Chicago. Chicago Journal. Volume 98, Issue 5.

Gómez, A. Beloz, J. Altern, J. (2001). El Botánica como una opción de atención médica culturalmente apropiada para los latinos.

Green, J. (1999). Conciencia Cultural en los Servicios Humanos. 3rd.ed. Englewood Cliffs, NJ. Prince Hall.

Hispanos en los Estados Unidos. (2006). Census Bureau, Population Estimates.

Heyck, D. (1994(. Barrios and borderlands: Cultures of Latinos and Latinas in the United States. New York: Routledge.

Insel, T. R. ((2008). Evaluación del costo económico de las enfermedades mentales graves. The American Journal of Psychiatry. 165 (6), 633-665.

Instituto Nacional de Salud Mental (2009-2012). Salud mental. NAMI Latino Multicultural Action Center.

Institute of Medicine (2003). The future of the publics' health in the 21st Century. The National Academies Press; Washington [Google Scholar]

John Hopkins-Medicine (2019). Psychiatry and Behavioral Sciences: The History of Psychiatric Social Work.

Kim, D. (1999). Práctica culturalmente de la competencia. Pacific Grove, CA: Books/Cole.

La comunidad hispana en el estado de Nueva York (2016). Thomas, P., DiNapoli, Contralor del estado de Nueva York. Casi uno de cada cinco neoyorquinos se identifica como hispano o latino.

Lewis, M. J., West, B., Bautista, L., Greenberg, A., Done-Pérez, I. (2005). Percepciones de los proveedores de servicios y los miembros de la comunidad sobre la violencia de pareja dentro de una comunidad latina. Educación para la salud y comportamiento. 32:69-83. (PubMed).

Lum, D. (1999). Práctica de competencia cultural. Pacific Grove, CA: Books/Cole.

Navarro Vásquez, C. (2014). Pew Research Center Analysis of Decennial Census and American Community Survey (IPUMS).

National Association of Social workers (2002). Code of Ethics of the National Association of Social Workers. Washington DC: Author.

Melville. L. M. (2012). On Culture.: Edward B. Tyler's Primitive Culture (1871). BRANCH: Britain, Representation and Ninteenth-Century History. Ed. Dino Franco Felluga. Extension of Romantisism and Victorianism on the Net. Web (2022).

Williams R. (1958). Culture and Society. Colunbia University Press.

National Association of Social Workers (2007). Definition of Clinical social Work. Washington DC: Autor.

National Association of Social Workers (2012). Clinical Social Work and Non-Clinical Social Work. Washington DC: Autor.

National Association of Social Workers (2014). NASW History of Psychiatric Social Work. Washington DC: Autor.

Nathan Kline Institute Center of Excellence in Culturally Competent Mental Health. (2019). Prácticas basadas en evidencia en apoyo de la competencia cultural en los servicios de salud mental.

National Association of Social Workers (2016). Standards of the NASW for the practice of social work on medical attention. Washington DC: Author.

Ortega, A. N., Rosenheck, R., Alegría, M. Desai, R. A. (2000). Aculturación y el riesgo de por vida de trastorno psiquiátrico y por uso de sustancias entre los hispanos. 188 (11); 728-35. PubMed.

Pew Research Center (2014). Analysis of Decennial Census and American Community Survey (IPUMS).

Porto Pérez, J., Merino, M. (2017-2019). Definición de Curandero. (https://definicion. de.curandero/).

Sue, D., Arredondo, P., McDavis, R. (1992). Multicultural counseling. Competencies and standards: a call to the profession. Journal of Counseling and Development, 70 (4), 477-486.

Uribe, R.M. Mora, O. L, Cortés, A. R. (2007). Voces del estigma. Percepción del estigma en pacientes y familias con enfermedad mental. Universitas Medica. 48 (3) Retrieved 8/12/2021.

Vega, W. A., López, S. R. (2001). Priority issues in Latino mental health services. Mental Health Research, Vol. 3, (4): 189-200. PubMed [Google Scholar]

Walker, S., Beckett, C. (2004-2005). Evaluación e Intervención de Trabajo Social. Russel House Publishing Company.

World Health Organization. (2014). Mental Health: A State of Wellbeing: Author.

Yeh, M., Hough, R., McCabe, K., Lau, A., Garland, A. (2004). Parental beliefs about the causes of child problems: Exploring racial/ethnic patterns. Journal of the American academy of Child and Adolescence Psychiatry, 43, 605-613.

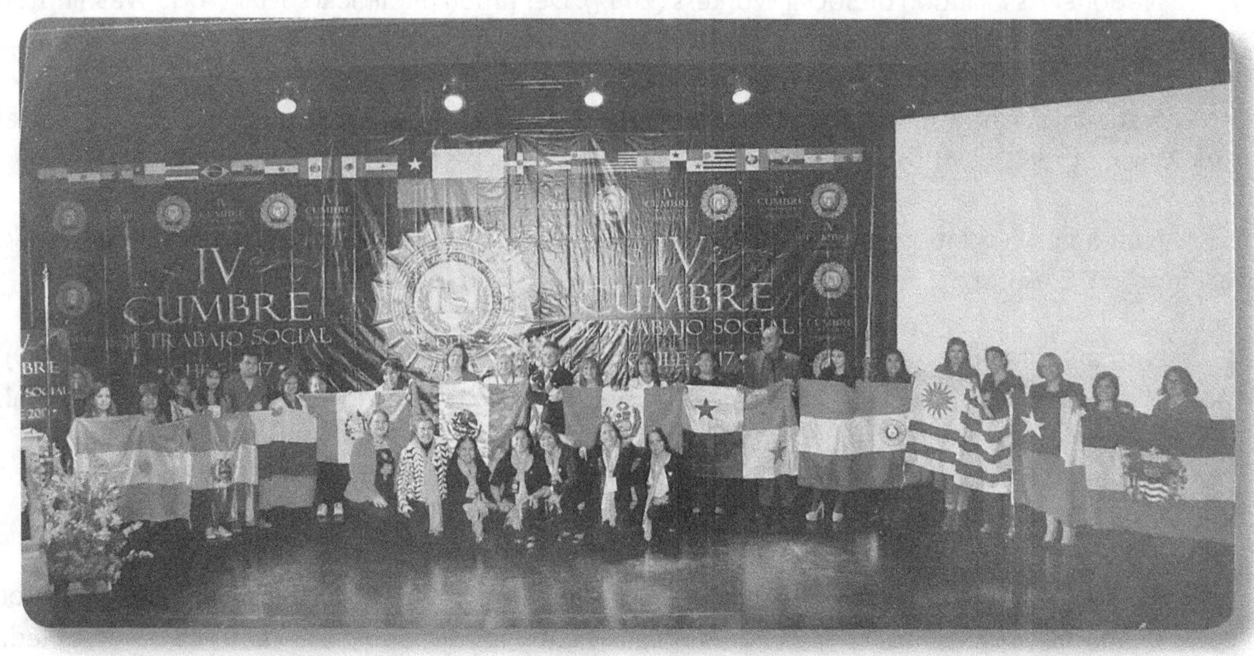

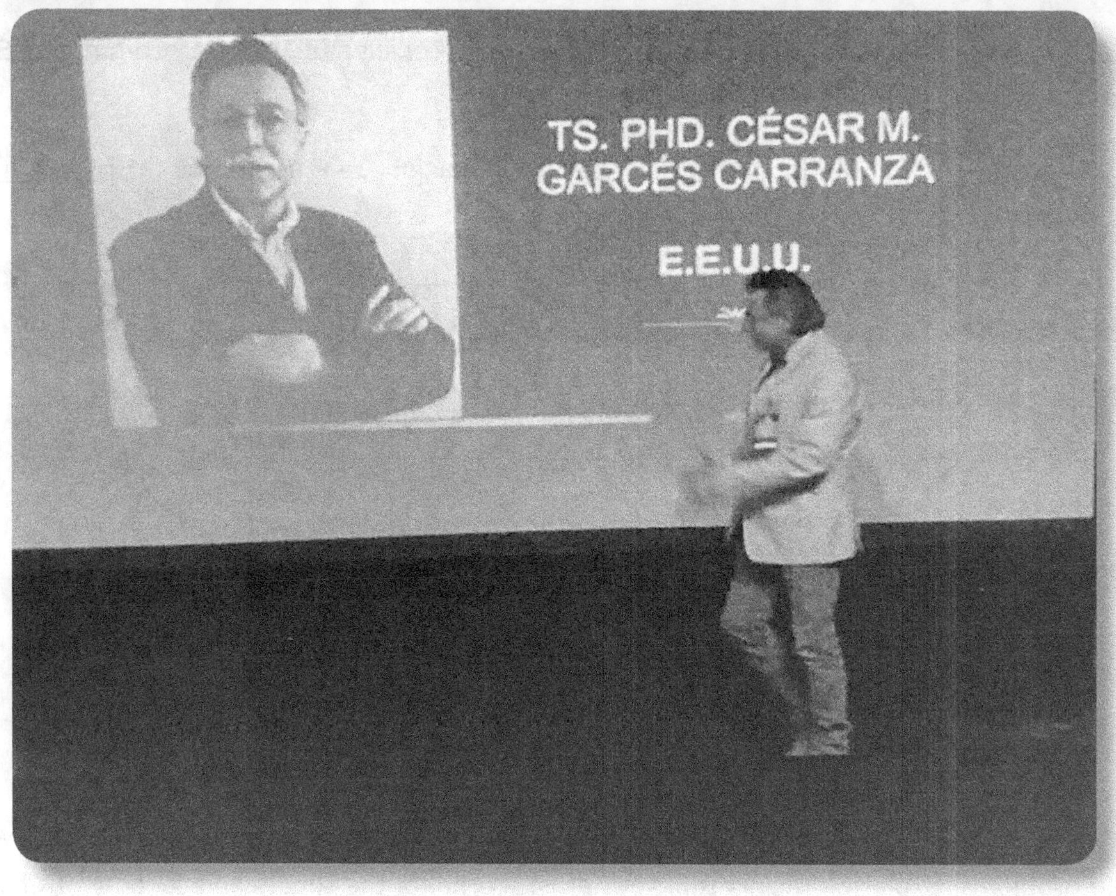
TS. PHD. CÉSAR M. GARCÉS CARRANZA
E.E.U.U.

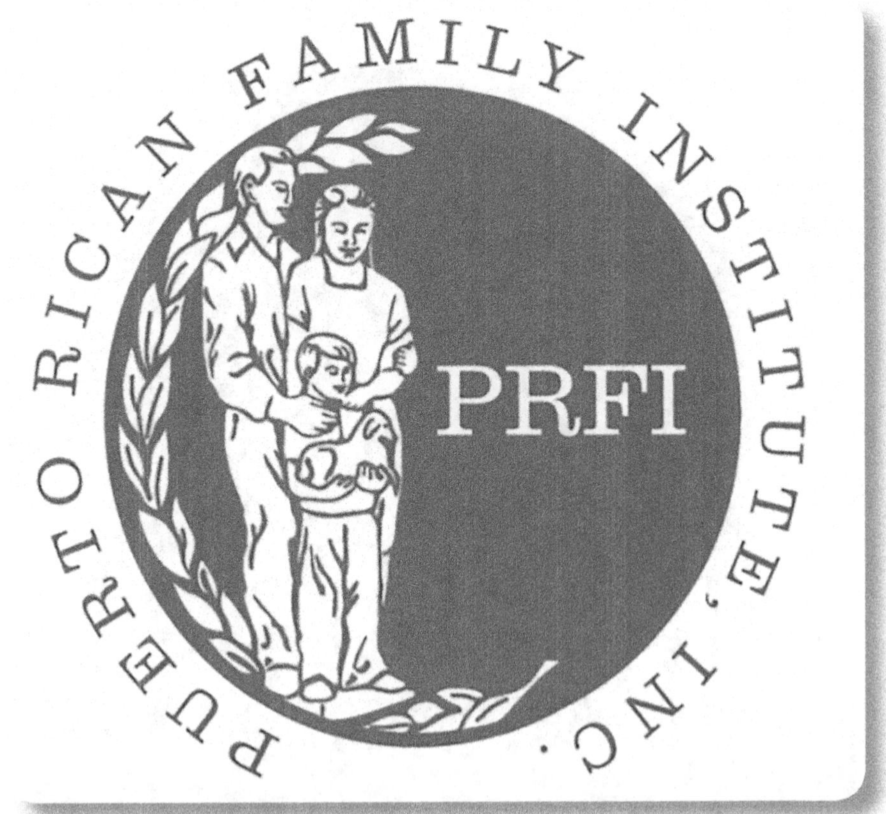
PUERTO RICAN FAMILY INSTITUTE, INC.
PRFI

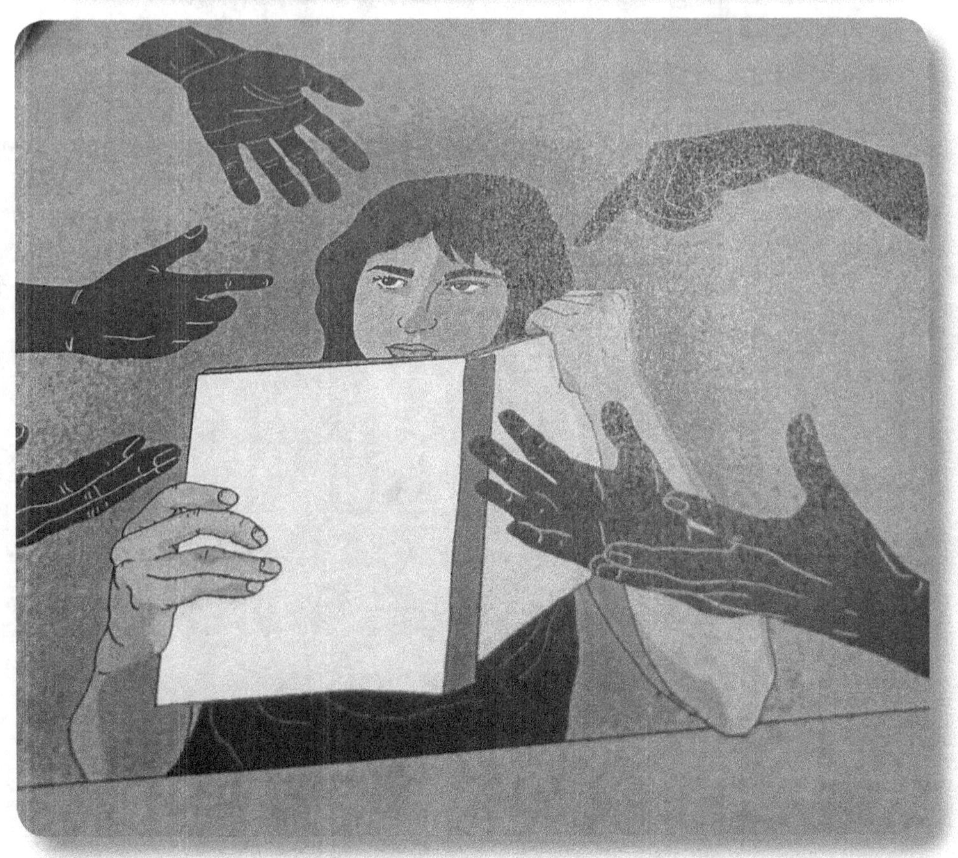

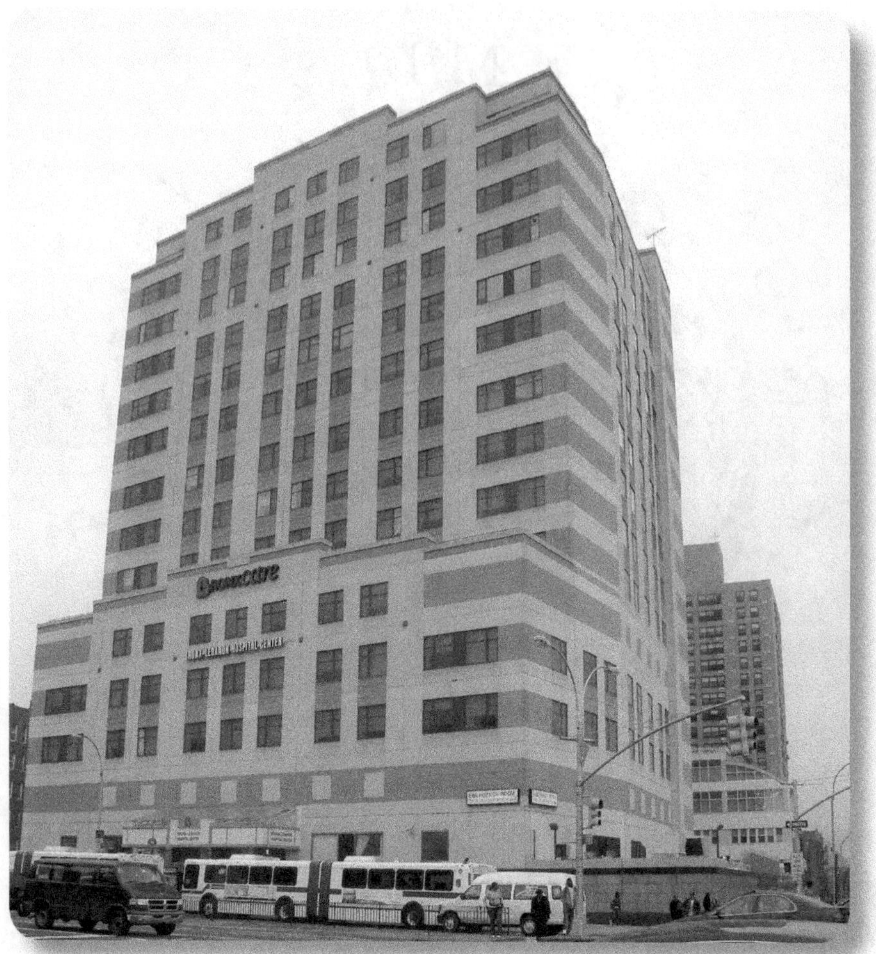

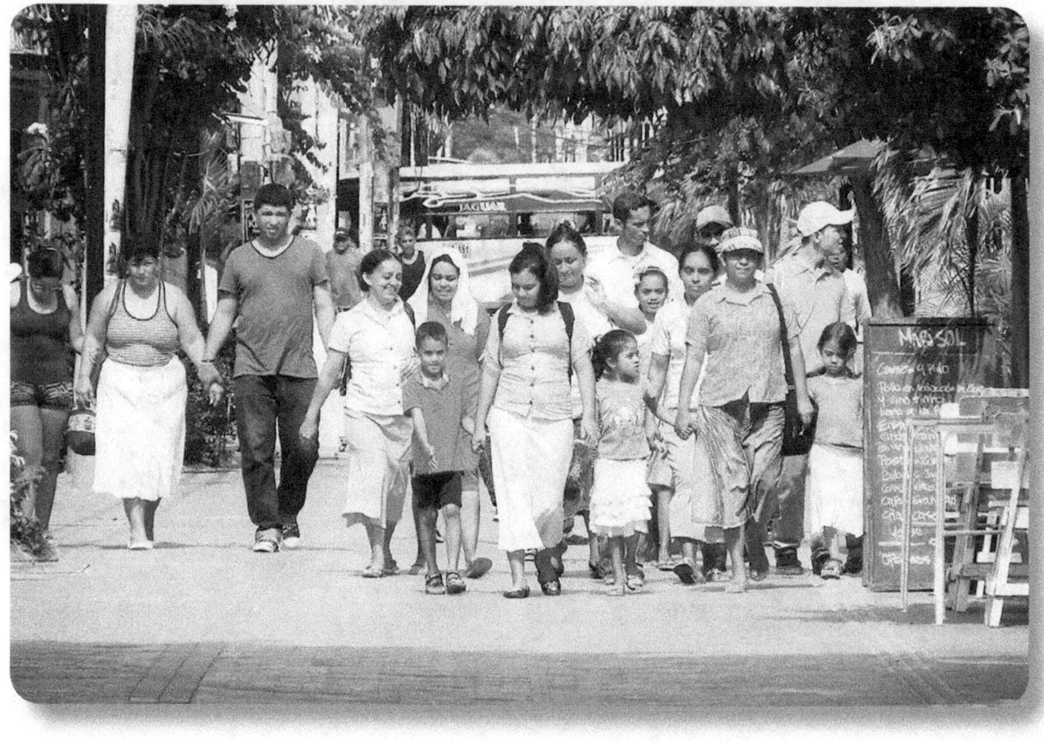

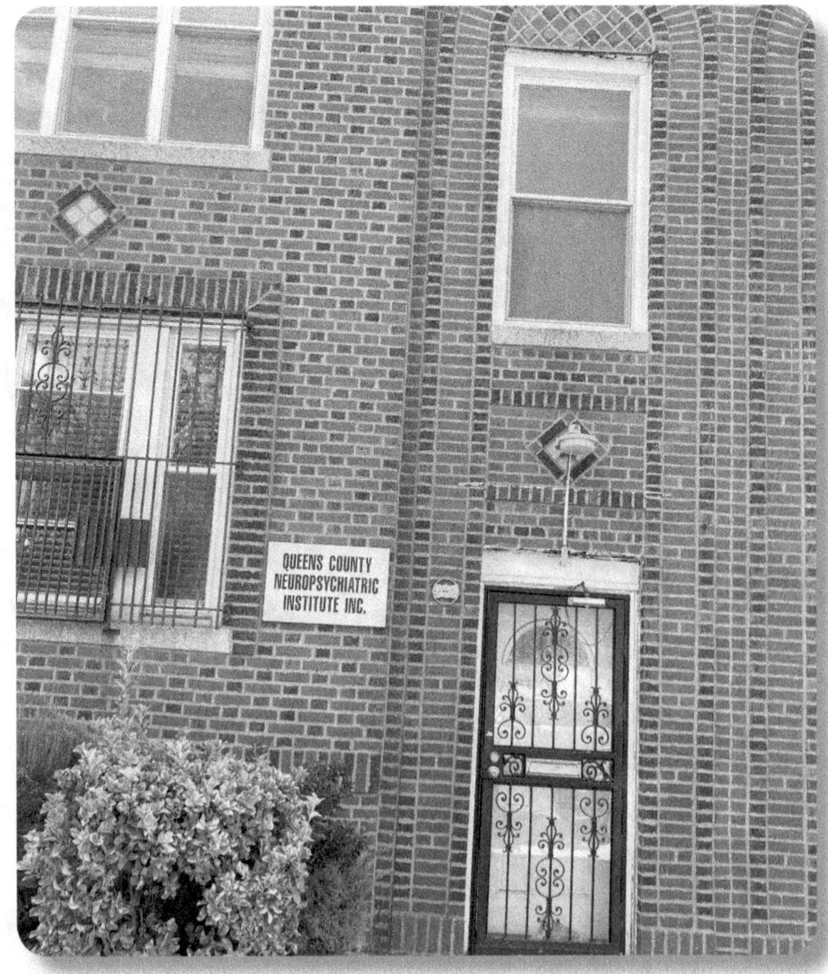
QUEENS COUNTY
NEUROPSYCHIATRIC
INSTITUTE INC.

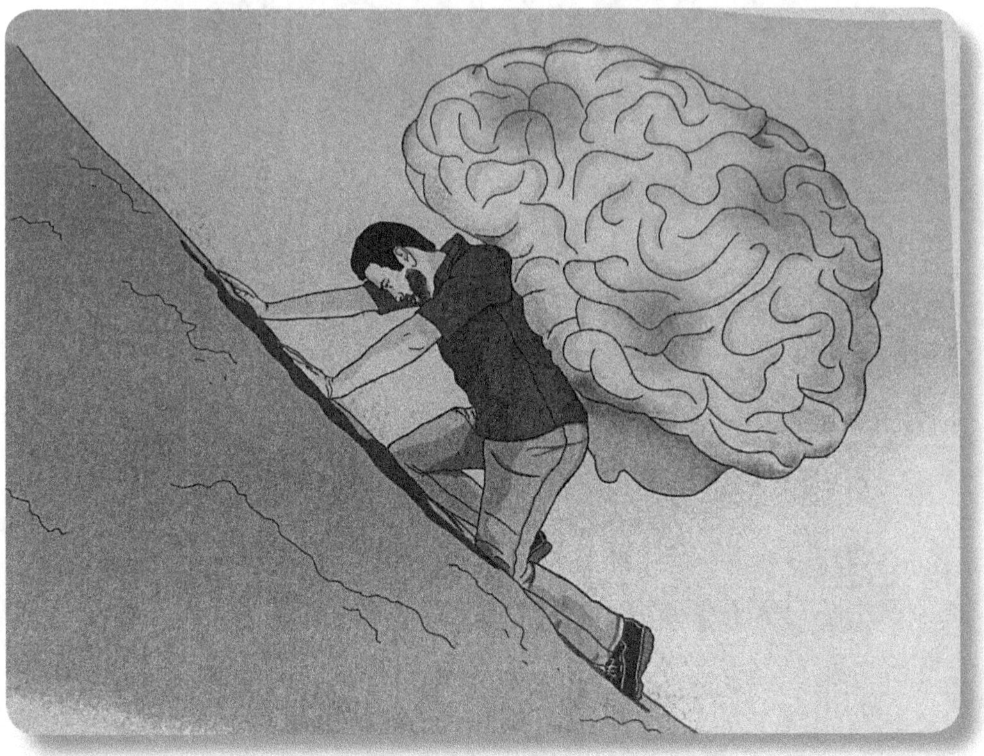

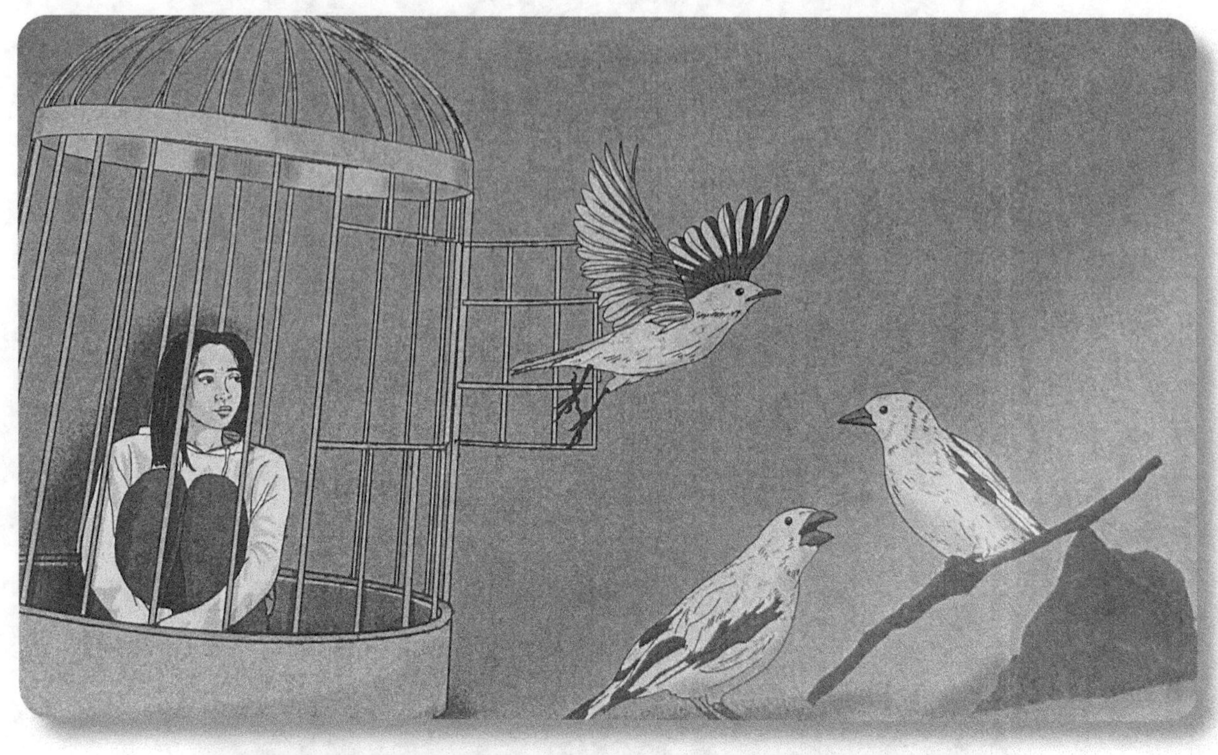

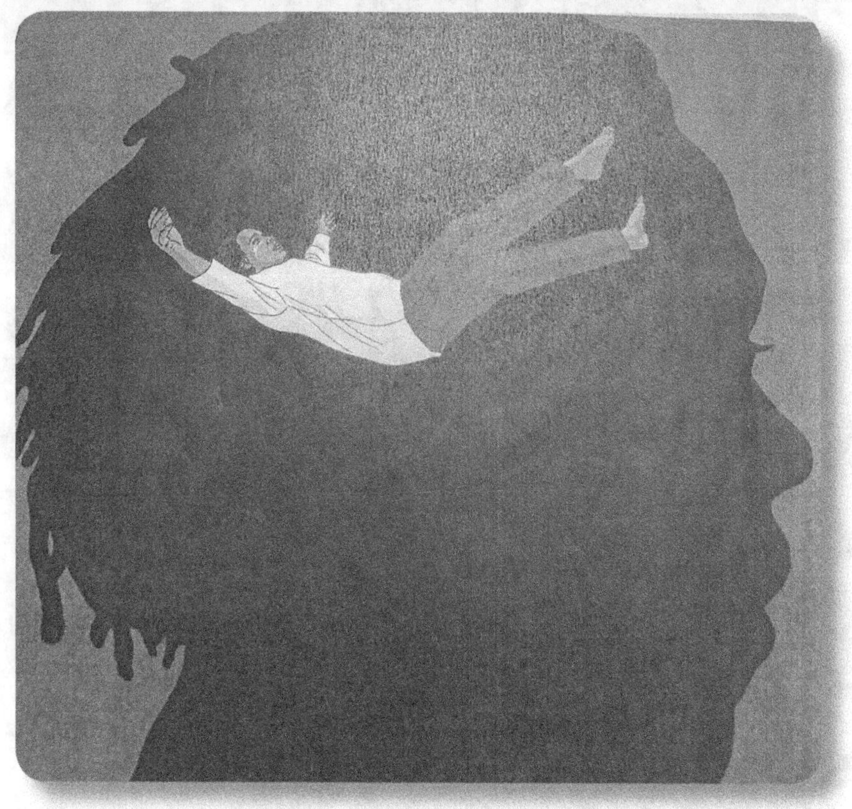

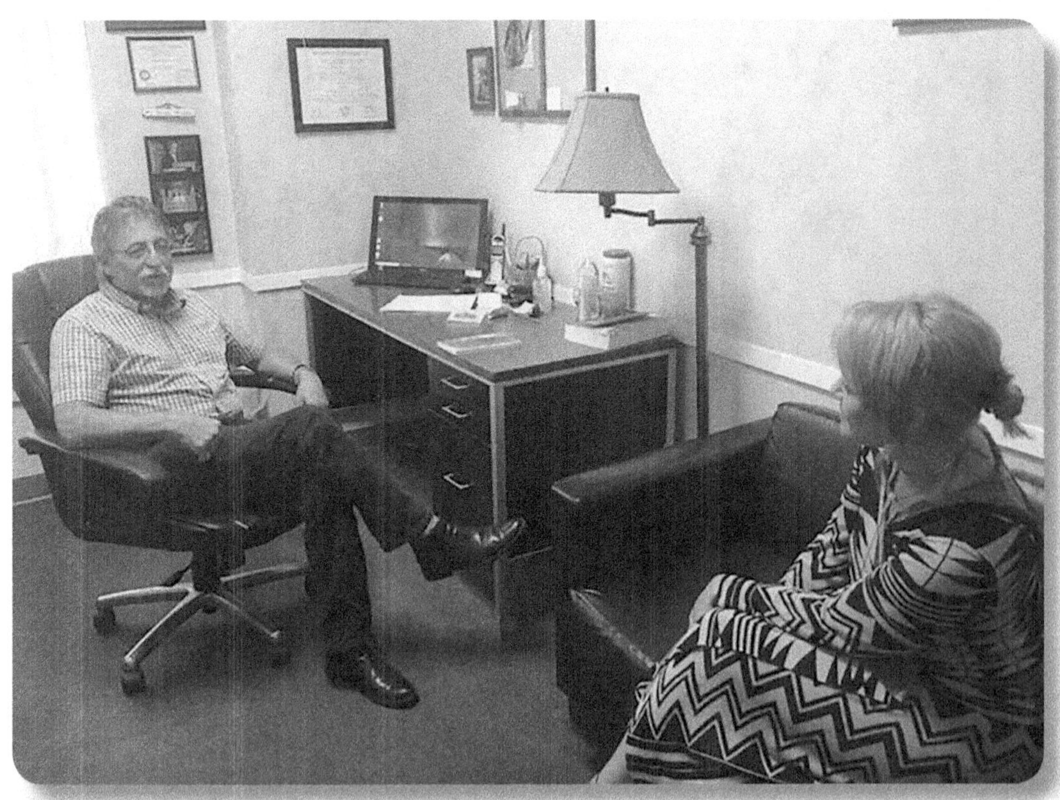

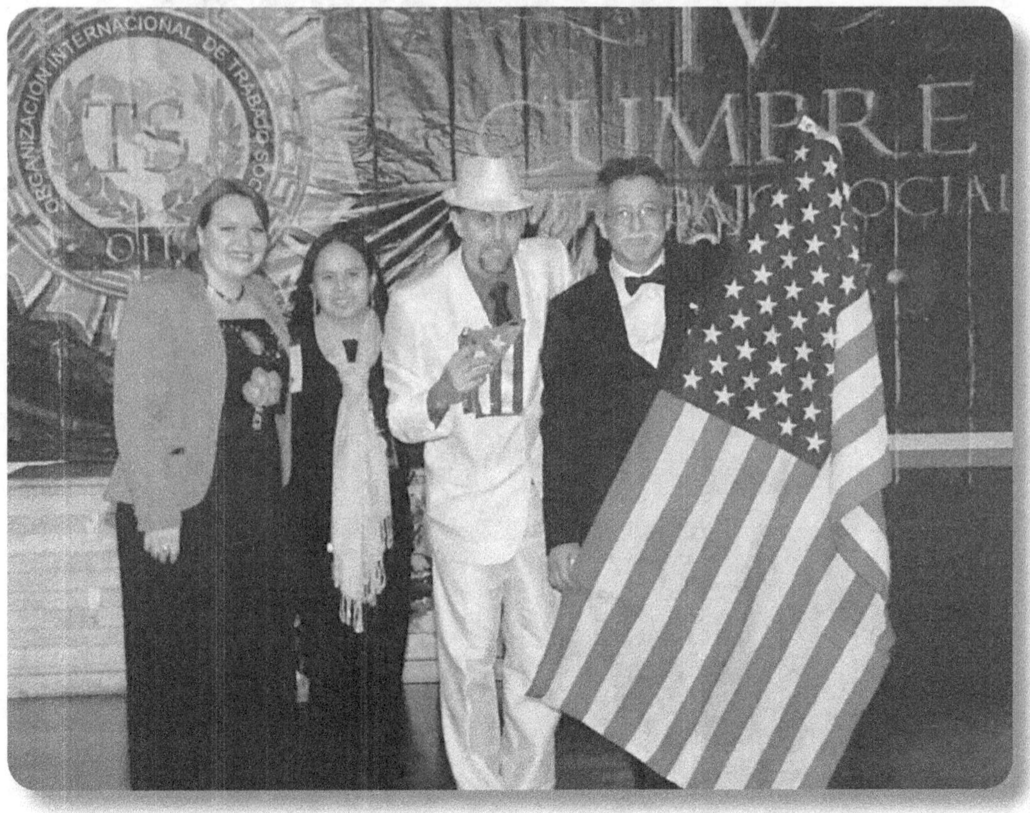
ORGANIZACION INTERNACIONAL DE TRABAJO SOCIAL
TS
OI
IV CUMBRE
TRABAJO SOCIAL

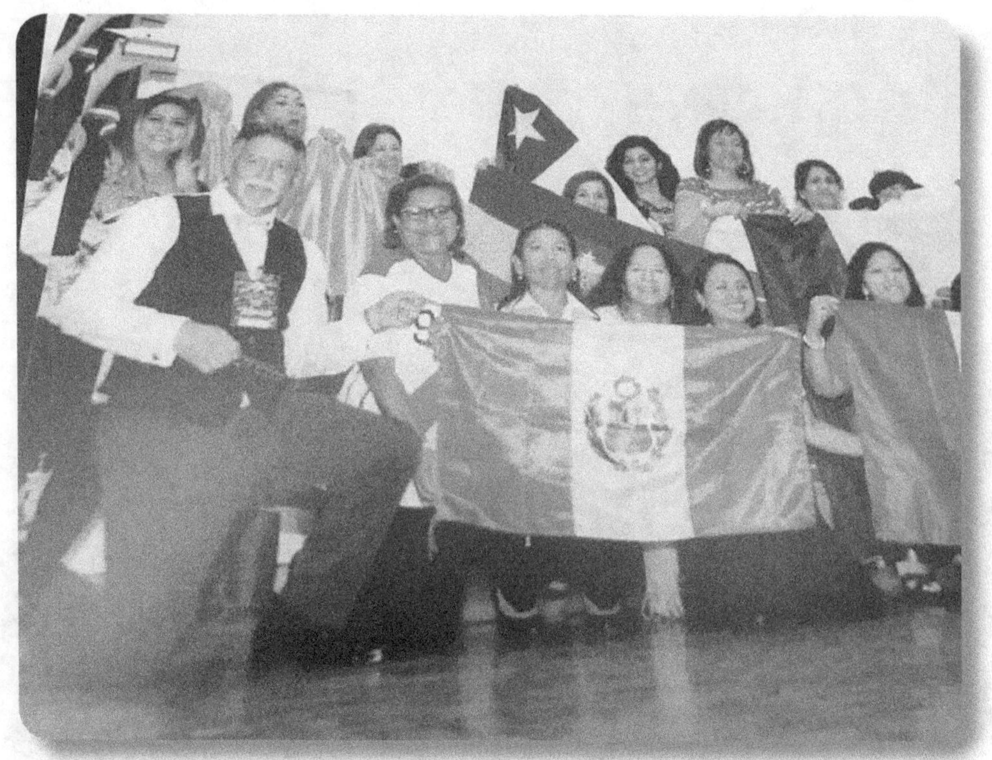

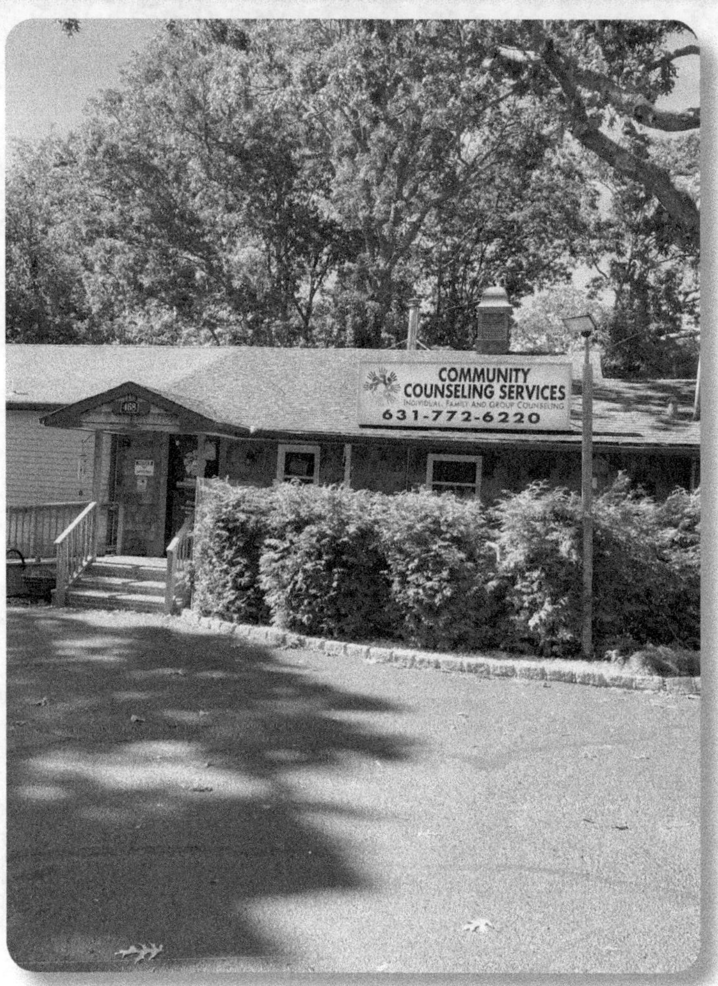
COMMUNITY
COUNSELING SERVICES
INDIVIDUAL, FAMILY AND GROUP COUNSELING
631-772-6220

www.ingramcontent.com/pod-product-compliance
Lightning Source LLC
Chambersburg PA
CBHW082248060726
47592CB00021B/3111